THE FAMILY GUIDE TO AROMATHERAPY

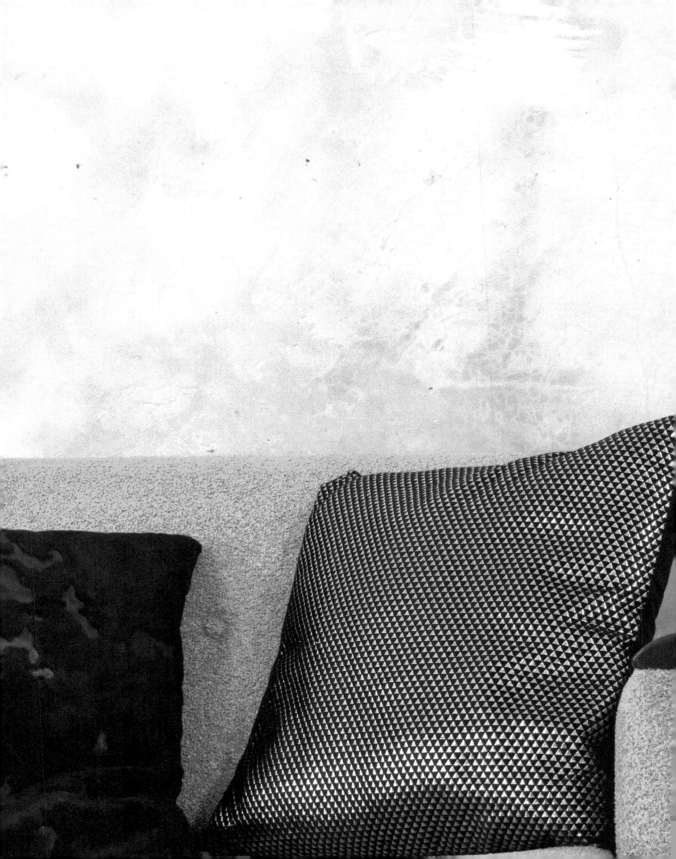

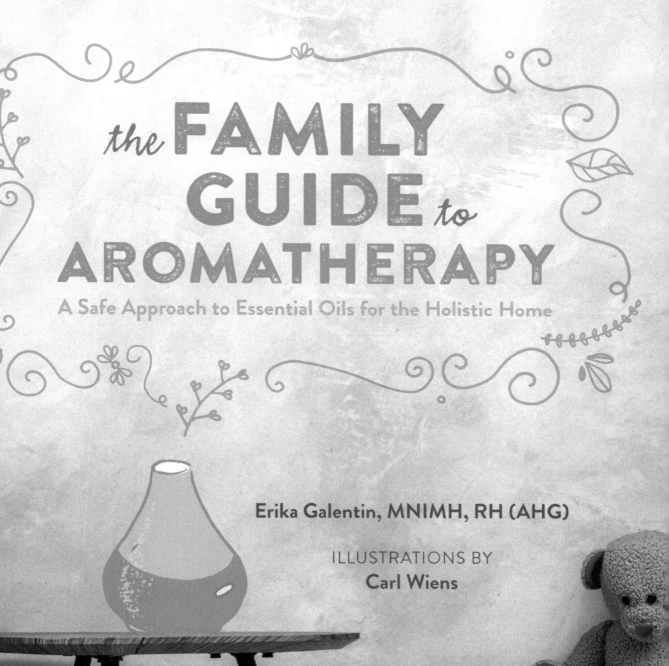

the FAMILY GUIDE to AROMATHERAPY

A Safe Approach to Essential Oils for the Holistic Home

Erika Galentin, MNIMH, RH (AHG)

ILLUSTRATIONS BY
Carl Wiens

ROCKRIDGE PRESS

To my husband, Nick; my daughters, Mary Grace and Olivia;
my business partner, Brooke; and my mother, Marion.
Thank you for your unwavering love and support.

Interior and Cover Designer: Emma Hall
Producer: Sue Bischofberger
Editor: Marisa A. Hines
Production Manager: Riley Hoffman
Production Editor: Melissa Edeburn

Illustration: © 2019 Carl Wiens/i2i Art Inc.

Photography: © Africa Studio/shutterstock, cover; © Naphat_Jorjee/shutterstock, cover; © Dionisvera /shutterstock, p. 128; © AmyLv/shutterstock, p. 129; © Kaiskynet Studio/shutterstock, p. 130; © Andrii Horulko/shutterstock, p. 131; © Scisetti Alfio/shutterstock, pp. 132, 139, 143; © Elena11/shutterstock, p. 133; © spline_x/shutterstock, pp. 134, 136, 145, 152, 153; © Anton-Burakov/shutterstock, p. 135; © azure1 /shutterstock, p. 137; © jiangdi/shutterstock, p. 138; © Igor Sirbu/shutterstock, p. 140; © MRAORAOR /shutterstock, p. 141; © Lotus Images/shutterstock, p. 142; © ELAKSHI CREATIVE BUSINESS/shutterstock, p. 144; © ansem/shutterstock, p. 146; © Superheang168/shutterstock, p. 147; © Maks Narodenko/shutterstock, pp. 148, 151; © Nattika/shutterstock, p. 149; © AmyLv/shutterstock, pp. 150, 154; © Anton Starikov/shutterstock, p. 155; © Elena Schweitzer/shutterstock, p. 156; © By Mark Brandon/shutterstock, p. 157.

ISBN: Print 978-1-64152-511-4 | eBook 978-1-64152-512-1

Contents

Introduction

One of my fondest childhood memories is the jovial aroma of a freshly cut Christmas tree wafting the magic of the season through our home. To this day, the scent of evergreen conifers, such as spruce, fir, and pine, carry me back in time to wintery holidays, a warm fireplace, freshly baked cookies, and spending time with my family in love and celebration. I also have spring and summer memories of working in the gardens with my mother and my sisters. When I close my eyes, I can still experience the pleasant scents of bright orange clusters of marigolds and vibrant red, juicy, ripe strawberries. These memories are very potent, and they all involve aroma produced by plants.

In fact, it was through aroma that I fell in love with plants and chose to dedicate my life to them. I was in my junior year of university when my roommate gifted me a book about essential oils and their long tradition of use in healing practices across the world. I couldn't have asked for a better and more appropriate birthday gift; I was three years into an undergraduate degree in medical anthropology, learning about how different cultures from around the world define health and disease and how they use plants to heal. It was the late '90s and essential oils were only just starting to hit the American market with gusto. I vividly remember the thrill of perusing the pages of that book and craving the opportunity to experience those powerful plant remedies firsthand.

By that time in my life, my exploration into the use of medicinal herbs for my own well-being had been limited to what I could find in books coupled with advice from the owner of a local herb shop. The Internet was not the information and shopping mecca it is now, and I was fortunate to have a place where I could go and a person with whom I could talk about buying herbs, like yarrow and chamomile, with which to experiment. One day I asked the shop owner if she would be willing to order some essential oils on my behalf, and much to my excitement, she agreed! Flipping through the pages of my beloved essential oil book, I chose rosemary to help stimulate my mind when, during the late hours of the evening, I would be stuck in the university library trying not to fall asleep. Clary sage was going to help me invoke a sense of calm in the face of exam jitters, and sweet marjoram was going to support my sense of well-being when I began to feel overwhelmed.

Cracking open my very first bottle of essential oil came with such an amazing sense of empowerment. I chose to open the rosemary first, and as I lowered my face to the small opening at the top of the bottle and gently breathed in through my nose, I was moved to tears of joy. I was overcome with the scent's uplifting strength, its sturdy character, and its motivational impact. What a blessing to have such tools for wellness right at my fingertips! In that moment I made a commitment to learn everything I possibly could about using herbs and essential oils to support human health and well-being. I had found my true heart path, one lined with these healing gifts from the plant kingdom.

After finishing my degree in anthropology, I was accepted into a medical degree program in Glasgow, Scotland, where I would learn human anatomy, physiology, pathology, and the clinical use of medicinal herbs and essential oils. Five intense and grueling years later, I would be calling myself a medical herbalist and clinical aromatherapist and would have a thriving clinical practice teaching my patients about how to use herbs and essential oils to achieve their wellness goals. Now, after more than a decade of clinical work, I am still as much in love with aromatherapy as I was with that first inhalation of rosemary. My sense of empowerment has only blossomed within this clinical environment as I witness on a daily basis the benefits that herbs and essential oils can provide to those who seek their guidance. Whether helping the weary get a good night's sleep or supporting the body through a viral infection, essential oils can improve the lives of both the very young and the very elderly when they are used safely and wisely.

My first experiences with essential oils were life changing but didn't come without some serious, and occasionally painful, trial and error. Unfortunately, those first bottles of essential oils did not arrive with an instruction manual, and there wasn't much information available about how to use them safely. Being an enthusiastic newbie, I made every safety mistake in the book; using undiluted essential oils in the bathtub led to some pretty serious chemical burns in some pretty delicate places. Luckily, I was experimenting only on myself and didn't end up harming others with my lack of understanding about the potent chemical nature of essential oils.

One of my biggest errors during these early self-experiments was believing that because essential oils are "natural" substances that come from plants, they are 100 percent safe, no matter how they are used. I learned quickly that this is not the case and am grateful that I, or anyone else, was not seriously harmed in the process. Unfortunately, even with all the knowledge about essential oils that exists today, which is so much more accessible than it was 20 years ago, the potential for harm has not abated. There are many horror stories about the inappropriate use of essential oils, enough to scare anyone away from bringing them into their homes and the lives of their loved ones.

Over a decade of clinical use combined with knowledge from a growing body of scientific research has helped me safely use essential oils to support the health and well-being of my clients, myself, and my beloved family. To safely use essential oils in your home, you won't need to earn a medical degree or to critically analyze scientific research papers (although reading research is always a good idea). You will need to apply some common sense and be willing to learn.

All you need to get started is a basic understanding of which essential oils are safe for the person using them and the appropriate dose and method of use for that specific person. Not all essential oils are appropriate for all people; infants and toddlers, young children, the elderly, pregnant and nursing mothers, and those who are seriously ill or taking pharmaceutical medications all require special consideration. In addition, methods of application and dose for the same essential oil will vary among these different groups of people in your family. You should always consult your midwife, pediatrician, doctor, or other licensed health care provider before using essential oils with these special populations. These experts may not always have all the answers to your questions, but they will be able to share their safety concerns for your consideration. Lastly, if you have pets in your home, understand that their bodies do not process chemical compounds like essential oils in the same ways that humans do; an essential oil that is deemed safe for even young toddlers may actually be toxic to your cat or dog. When using essential oils in your home, you will need to be sure that your pets are not being unduly exposed and that you consult with your veterinarian and do your research before attempting to use essential oils near your pets.

Another key to safety is having realistic expectations. As a medical herbalist, I am always surprised when I read claims that herbs or essential oils can "prevent," "treat," or "cure" medical problems. Such claims are akin to using essential oils as if they were pharmaceuticals. Although essential oils can have incredibly powerful actions, they have not been studied and tested with the same scientific rigor as pharmaceuticals and are not nearly as legally regulated. Therefore, claiming that essential oils can prevent, treat, or cure anything is not only unsafe; it is both unlawful and beyond our current scope of understanding. Yes, there have been magnificent leaps and bounds in the use of essential oils to counter bacteria and other infection-causing organisms, and yes, there is an increasing body of research that verifies the use of essential oils in numerous health care scenarios. However, I am of the opinion that it is not only safer but also more effective to shift our perspectives about the role of essential oils in our overall wellness strategies away from preventing, treating, or curing medical problems. Instead, we should aim to understand how essential oils may assist our minds and bodies as we confront these medical problems. For example, instead of thinking about how to use essential oils to treat your anxiety symptoms, you would instead explore the use of essential oils that may help you relax and focus on your breath. Think of essential oils as tools for wellness, not as treatments for symptoms or disease.

Realistic expectations of aromatherapy are also derived from the understanding of what essential oils are and how they are produced. The essential oil of a plant, also known as the *volatile oil*, represents a specific type of chemical family. However, within the plant of origin, that oil represents just one of multiple chemical families. The medicinal properties of an herb, for example yarrow or chamomile, may or may not be present in the essential oil; they may result from other chemical compounds that do not make it into the essential oil when it is extracted. Consider frankincense essential oil and the claims that it can treat cancer. Boswellic acid, found in frankincense resin, has demonstrated anticancer properties in laboratory and animal studies. However, boswellic acid does not exist in the essential oil, and therefore, the essential oil cannot be said to have these same properties.

Maintaining realistic expectations of aromatherapy can also provide us with a prudent and intentional approach to the use of essential oils. Not only does this approach keep our actions focused on safety, but it also invites core concepts of a holistic practice into our homes: sustainability and environmental responsibility. For every gallon of essential oil produced, hundreds and sometimes thousands of pounds of plant material are either cultivated or harvested from the wild. Essential oils require a lot of natural resources to produce, and as mindful and responsible consumers, we should hold this truth in our minds and hearts with every drop we use.

In closing, approaching aromatherapy for the first time can feel scary and overwhelming. After all, we want what is best for our families and we want to keep them safe from harm. However, I want you to feel as empowered and excited as I did with that first bottle of rosemary essential oil, knowing that with the practical advice presented in this book, you will have a clear road map to get you started on your aromatherapy journey. It has been a real joy putting all of this information together for you in one place for a strong foundation of safe practices. As you embark on this rewarding path, there are a few key tenets to remember: Everyone is different and will respond to aromatherapy in different ways, *more* does not equate to *more effective*, and the old adage "a little goes a long way" absolutely rings true.

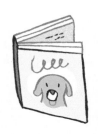
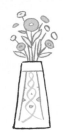
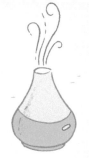

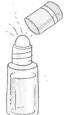
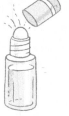
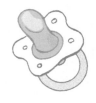
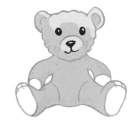
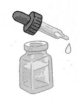
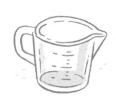
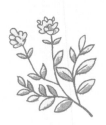
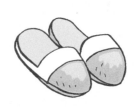
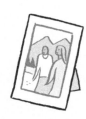
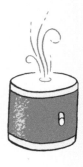

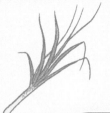

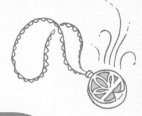

AROMATHERAPY PRACTICES, SAFE BLENDS, AND GUIDELINES FOR YOUR FAMILY

In Part I of this book, we will explore aromatherapy practices, safety guidelines, and essential oil blends for different members of your family. We begin with a review of the benefits of aromatherapy and an introduction to safety guidelines for the use of essential oils. The subsequent chapters provide a focused approach to working with family members of different age groups. Part I concludes with ways to incorporate essential oils into the general care and cleaning of your household.

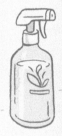
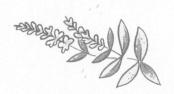

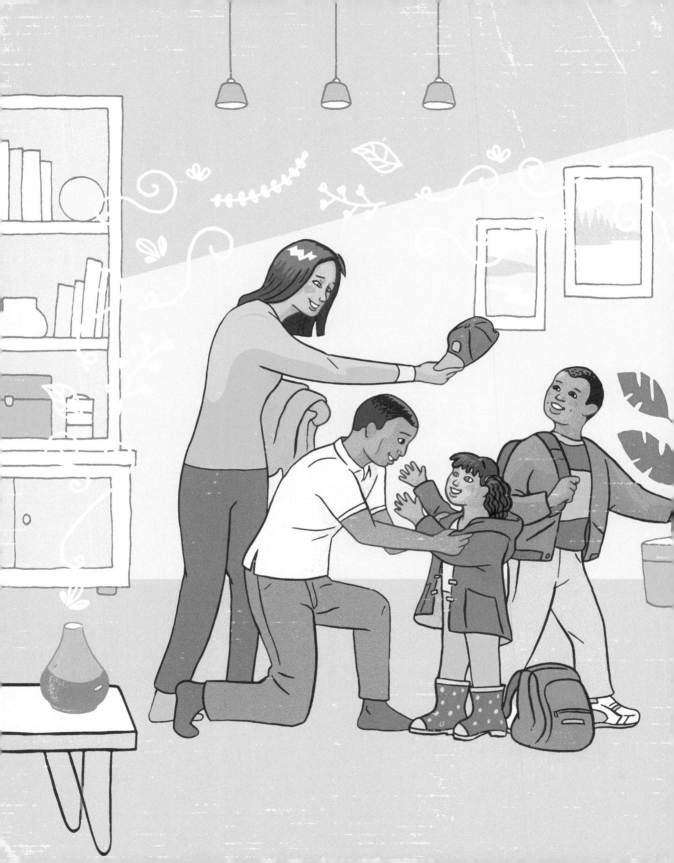

Chapter One

INTRODUCTION TO AROMATHERAPY

What Is Aromatherapy?

Plants have always played a fundamental role in human health and well-being. They provide the nutrients necessary for the growth and vitality of the body as well as produce hundreds of medicinal compounds that can support its healthy functioning. Today, plants' healing properties have been captured and concentrated in the form of pharmaceuticals, dietary supplements, and essential oils.

Essential oils, also known as volatile oils, are a family of medicinal compounds extracted from plants that are often responsible for the aroma of a plant as well as its flavor. For example, essential oils are largely responsible for the scent and taste of our most beloved culinary herbs, such as basil, mint, and rosemary. Within the plant, these powerful compounds provide protection and promote survival of the plant by attracting pollinators and warding off predators and disease.

In their extracted and concentrated form, essential oils serve as the principal tools of the practice of aromatherapy. Through both traditional use and scientific research, essential oils have been shown to be capable of providing significant support to many aspects of the human body, including our nervous, immune, respiratory, circulatory, integumentary (skin), genitourinary, and digestive systems. They can also be considered allies to our emotional well-being; aroma from essential oils can invoke significant shifts in the human mind and psyche, providing assistance as we traverse our emotional experiences. As you will discover, aromatherapy can be incredibly supportive to the health and well-being of your entire family.

In the following sections, we will be exploring core safety guidelines and best practices for using essential oils on and around your loved ones. Incorporating the safe practice of aromatherapy into your home is achieved through making informed choices about which essential oils to use as well as their appropriate doses and methods of application. These choices will be dependent upon differences between family members, including their age, health status, and wellness goals. Not all essential oils will be appropriate for all members of your family. As you explore the benefits of aromatherapy in your home, it is important that you continue to research the essential oils you choose to use. In fact, it is best practice to master a few really versatile essential oils, instead of accumulating a plethora of highly specific oils that you know very little about.

Introduction to Essential Oil Guidelines

ESSENTIAL OILS TO AVOID

TOXIC	Ajowan • Bitter almond • Boldo • Buchu • Calamus • Camphor (brown and yellow) • Horseradish • Mustard • Rue • Sassafras • Tansy • Thuja • Wormseed • Wormwood
HAZARDOUS	Bitter fennel • Cassia • Garlic • Hyssop • Mugwort • Onion • Pennyroyal • Sage • Santolina • Savory • Spanish lavender (*L. stoechas*) • Sweet birch • Wintergreen
SKIN IRRITANTS & SENSITIZERS	Bay (*Pimenta racemosa*) • Cinnamon bark and leaf • Citronella • Clove bud • Cumin • Inula • Lemon verbena • Lemongrass • Oregano • Oxidized oils from the pine, cypress, and citrus families • Tagetes • Thyme • Ylang-ylang
PHOTOSENSITIZERS	Angelica root • Bergamot • Bitter orange – expressed • Cumin • Grapefruit • Lemon – expressed • Lemongrass • Lime – expressed • Melissa
ENDANGERED, THREATENED, OR VULNERABLE SPECIES	Agarwood • Atlas cedarwood • Elemi • Frankincense (*Boswellia sacra*) • Guaiac wood • Guggul • Hemlock spruce • Juniper • Opopanax • Palo santo • Rosewood • Sandalwood • Spikenard

Safe Practices

Even though essential oils are derived from plants and provide many wonderful wellness benefits, it is important to approach all essential oils with caution. As highly concentrated and potent chemical compounds, essential oils that are used inappropriately can cause adverse reactions, particularly when used on and around sensitive loved ones, including babies, young children, the elderly, and even your pets. In addition, essential oils that are deemed safe even for the most sensitive of individuals can actually become irritating or toxic if used in high doses or for prolonged periods of time. In a process referred to as *sensitization*, repeated and prolonged exposure to the same essential oil can lead to increased sensitivity and likelihood for adverse reactions to that specific essential oil. However, most essential oils are considered safe for home use and pose a very limited risk for harm when basic safety guidelines are followed.

Several factors can influence the safety of essential oils, including the quality and purity of the essential oil, the chemical composition of that oil, and its dose and method of application. Unfortunately, high quality and purity cannot always be assumed. In fact, many essential oils on the market today are commonly adulterated with both natural and synthetic contaminants. Essential oils that have been adulterated are much more likely to cause adverse toxicity reactions, including chemical burns and skin reactions. Later in this chapter, you will find useful tips about how to vet essential oils for quality and purity.

Even if pure and of high quality, some essential oils pose a greater risk of adverse reactions than others. This potential for risk grows with internal use of essential oils, a practice that is not recommended unless you are working with a qualified health care practitioner. Adverse reactions are less likely with the external applications covered in this book. For example, there is a very limited risk of adverse reactions to essential oils with the appropriate use of aromatherapy diffusers. The safety risks for topical application of essential oils may include mild to severe skin reactions, such as contact dermatitis or chemical burns, and photosensitization (when an essential oil increases your risk of sunburn). The likelihood of these adverse skin reactions is based upon the chemical makeup of the essential oil, whether or not it has become oxidized (gone off), how it was produced (expressed, steam distilled, or solvent extracted), the dose and dilution being used, and the integrity of the skin. Wounded, diseased, or inflamed skin may be more sensitive to essential oils and therefore more likely to elicit sensitization or adverse reactions. Risk for sensitization, irritation, and other adverse skin reactions is also more likely when using undiluted essential oils.

There are varying opinions among aromatherapy practitioners about whether or not essential oils should be used directly on the skin without diluting them in a base or carrier oil (see Application Guidelines, page 7). However, dilution is the best way to keep your practice of aromatherapy safe and to avoid sensitization and adverse skin reactions. If you have sensitive skin or are using essential oils with infants, toddlers, children under 12, or the elderly, you should always dilute essential oils before applying them topically. In addition, if you are introducing an essential oil for the first time to anyone in your family, you have the option of performing a patch test. Although not a 100 percent guarantee of safety, patch testing may help you determine whether or not an individual may have an underlying sensitivity or allergy to a specific essential oil before applying it to large areas of the skin.

To perform a patch test, add the essential oil to the appropriate amount of carrier oil depending on the dilution ratio recommended for the person you are testing (see Application Guidelines, below). Never use undiluted essential oils for patch testing. Place 1 to 2 drops of this dilution on the inner forearm or inner elbow and cover with a bandage for 24 hours, periodically checking for reactions. Make sure that the area does not get wet during the test. If any immediate irritation or adverse reaction occurs, remove the bandage and wash the area with soap and water. If after 24 to 48 hours from removal of the bandage no reaction has occurred, it is likely that the diluted essential oil can be used safely on the skin. However, if redness is present and accompanied by itching, burning, swelling, or the development of blisters, it is likely that a sensitivity or allergy to that essential oil is occurring, and it shouldn't be used.

Application Guidelines

Each chapter in this book has been dedicated to specific age groups and stages of life and includes appropriate dosing and dilution recommendations as well as essential oil blends that are considered safe for each group. To be clear, suggestions and recommendations for essential oil use covered in this book are referring to external use of essential oils only; ingesting essential oils or inserting them into body cavities, such as the mouth, nose, ears, vagina, or anus, is not recommended unless you are working with a qualified health care practitioner.

Methods of safe external use covered in this book include aromatic (through diffusion and inhalation) and topical (diluted application to the skin using a carrier or base). These methods are the most common in external use and, when approached appropriately, constitute a very low risk for adverse events.

DOSING AND DILUTION FOR TOPICAL APPLICATION

Diluting an essential oil or essential oil blend simply means combining it with a carrier or base for topical application to the skin. Usually expressed as a percentage, dilution ratios can be easily converted to the number of drops of an essential oil that should be used per volume or weight measurement of a carrier or base. This percentage or number of drops will vary depending on the potency of the essential oil and the age of the person it is being applied to. Each chapter provides recommended dilutions for the respective age group covered in that chapter. It is important to note that dilution ratios used for topical applications may not necessarily translate to aromatic applications, such as diffusion and personal inhalers.

CARRIERS AND BASES

Carriers or bases can include a variety of substances, including vegetable and nut oils, such as coconut or olive oil; herbal-infused oils, such as calendula; or lotions and creams. It is important to note that vegetable, nut, and herbal-infused oils are not essential oils. Other common carriers include aloe vera gel, unscented liquid soaps, shampoos, and body washes. Other substances, such as cosmetic clay or Epsom salt, are also often used as bases, but essential oils should always first be diluted with a carrier oil before being mixed with these dry ingredients.

WATER AND ESSENTIAL OILS

Water or a waterlike substance, such as vinegar or witch hazel extract, is not a reliable choice as a carrier or base for topical application. Oil and water don't mix, and when adding essential oils to water or waterlike substances, you will notice that the essential oil will eventually collect and float on the surface. For this reason, it is suggested not to put essential oils into a bath without diluting them in a carrier oil first; similarly, essential oils should never be added to drinking water or other beverages as flavoring agents. In both these situations, the essential oil will not disperse throughout the water but rather will remain in its concentrated form on the surface, causing an increased likelihood of adverse reactions as a result of direct, undiluted exposure to sensitive areas of skin or mucous membranes.

Water is used to dilute essential oils for diffusion and when making mists or sprays for cleaning and air freshening. If using sprays or mists, you will need to shake them vigorously in order to temporarily disperse the essential oil into them. Spraying aromatherapy mists onto the skin or face or in the eyes is not recommended.

DIRECT INHALATION

Direct inhalation, whether using a personal aromatherapy inhaler, smelling a drop on a facial tissue or cotton swab, or just sniffing the open bottle, can be the quickest and most personal way to use essential oils. This method is handy to use while traveling, when needing acute support, or when you are in a public space and wish to be respectful to those around you by not inadvertently exposing them to essential oils without their consent. Using essential oils in this way for direct inhalation can be intense, and if using a facial tissue or a cotton swab, 1 drop of essential oil should suffice. It is best to avoid direct contact with the sensitive tissues of your nasal passages. You should restrict your exposure to only a few inhalations over 5 to 10 minutes, and then take a break, repeating as needed several times a day.

It is not advised to use the open bottle, inhaler, or tissue method with babies and young children. If, however, you choose to allow children to interact with essential oils in this way, be mindful of their response, and if they pull away, do not force their exposure. The same goes for the elderly and those who cannot communicate discomfort or discontent. It is best to not let children handle open bottles of essential oil. If using the inhaler or tissue method, do not leave children unattended, and ensure that contact with the mouth, nasal cavity, and eyes is avoided.

DIFFUSION

Diffusion uses a device to distribute essential oil molecules through the air. These devices come in a variety of forms, and the amount of essential oil that should be used in a diffuser will likely be based on the manufacturer's instructions. Be sure to read through these instructions carefully and follow their recommendations. In addition, some oils are more potent than others and will need to be used in smaller amounts. You will also want to ensure proper air flow through a room where individuals or pets are playing or resting. Being trapped in a room with strong aromas, even if from essential oils, can lead to toxicity reactions, including headaches, nausea, and dizziness, as well as allergy-like symptoms, such as runny nose, burning and watery eyes, and difficulty breathing.

The FDA and Essential Oils

It is important to note that at the time of writing, essential oils and the essential oil market are not regulated by the Food and Drug Administration (FDA). Therefore, claims about the use of essential oils in the prevention, treatment, and curing of symptoms and disease are unlikely to have been evaluated by the FDA and, as such, are unlawful. In addition, purity and quality of essential oils are also not regulated by the FDA or any other oversight organization. In fact, there is no regulatory definition for the term *essential oil*. At this time, it is up to manufacturers to supply quality and purity evidence to consumers at their discretion. Lastly, you may encounter discussions about the safety of internal use of essential oils based on the oil in question being listed on the FDA's "Generally Recognized as Safe" list. This list is intended for food manufacturers, and essential oils on this list are considered safe only as additives to food-flavoring products. Being present on this list does not indicate that the essential oil is safe for internal medicinal use. For more information, consult the following:

✦ https://www.fda.gov/Cosmetics/ProductsIngredients/Products/ucm127054.htm

✦ https://www.fda.gov/Cosmetics/ProductsIngredients/Ingredients/ucm388821 .htm#essential

✦ https://www.fda.gov/Food/IngredientsPackagingLabeling/GRAS/default.htm

SAFETY TIPS

✦ Do not use essential oils internally or place into body cavities unless you are working with a qualified health care practitioner.

✦ Do not use essential oils as flavoring agents for foods or beverages.

✦ Avoid using essential oils undiluted on the skin or in the bath.

✦ Avoid letting essential oils come in contact with mucous membranes and sensitive tissues, like the eyes. If contact occurs, wash with water, and if irritation persists, seek medical care.

✦ Wash hands after use. Wear gloves when using cleaning supplies made with essential oils.

✦ Avoid the use of essential oils that are known to be hazardous or known to cause sensitization, irritation, or increased photosensitivity.

✦ Avoid essential oils produced from plants that you might be allergic to. For example, if you have an allergy to plants in the daisy/aster (*Asteraceae*) family, it is best to avoid essential oils from plants in that family.

✦ Do not expose skin to sunlight or ultraviolet lamps for 12 to 18 hours after applying essential oils with known photosensitizing properties, including homemade insect repellents and skin care products.

✦ One dilution does not fit all! Do your research before assuming.

✦ Prolonged exposure and excessive use of essential oils can lead to irritation and sensitization and, in some cases, systemic toxicity.

BEST PRACTICES

+ Consult with your qualified health care provider before using essential oils on yourself or your family members. If interested in using essential oils to help your pets, be sure to do your research first and consult with your veterinarian before trying them.

+ Listen to your body and the bodies of your loved ones and what they are communicating about an essential oil interaction. "Detox" reactions are a farce and are more likely to be a symptom of a severe adverse reaction.

+ Take breaks. Although it is generally considered safe to diffuse essential oils daily or use a personal inhaler several times a day, it is highly recommended that you give yourself, your family, and your wallet a break from time to time.

+ Keep essential oils in closed containers away from heat and light. Make sure to label your blends properly; include all ingredients and the date the blend was made on the label.

+ Keep essential oils away from the reach of children and pets. Most poisonings from essential oils have been accidental and have occurred because children gained access to and ingested open containers of essential oils. If accidental ingestion occurs, call poison control and seek medical care. Be sure to bring the bottle with you.

+ Do not purchase essential oils produced from endangered, threatened, or vulnerable plant species.

+ Remember that aromatherapy is a journey, not a destination. Always strive to expand your knowledge through research. Keep a journal of what has worked, what hasn't, what you might do differently, and your favorite blends and recipes.

SHOPPING FOR ESSENTIAL OILS

Buying essential oils can be intimidating, as there are so many companies and brands to choose from. It's always a good idea to research a company before you purchase its products. Does it have good customer reviews? Does it have sound sustainability and environmental policies? Is it making unlawful claims about how its essential oils can prevent, treat, or cure symptoms or disease?

If shopping online, it is sometimes best to avoid third-party sellers and to focus on sourcing your essential oils directly from the company that produces them to ensure accountability. The company's website should list both the common and scientific names of the essential oils as well as the part of the plant the oil came from (e.g., leaves, flowers, roots, fruits). The website should also list the country of origin.

In their enthusiasm for their products, essential oil companies may use decorative marketing language. There are common marketing terms, such as "certified therapeutic grade," that reflect a company's belief in the quality and purity of its essential oils. However, be aware that there is no external oversight or grading system for essential oil purity or quality, and terms such as "certified therapeutic grade" are based on internal measures only. Although there are no tests that can guarantee that an essential oil is 100 percent free from adulterants or contaminants, most reputable companies will provide the results of analytical tests they have completed themselves. The most common of these purity tests is the gas chromatography/mass spectrometry assay (GCMS), the report of which you should be able to see or download from the company's website. This information can instill consumer confidence.

Always read labels and carefully inspect the ingredient list. Most bottles should contain only 100 percent pure essential oil; however, expensive essential oils, such as rose, melissa, neroli, or jasmine, may come prediluted in vegetable or nut oil, which should be indicated on the label and in the ingredient list. Bottles labeled *fragrance oil*, *perfume oil*, or *identical oil* are not essential oils and should not be considered such. The label should also include both the common and scientific names of the plant the oil is extracted from. It may list the part of the plant used (e.g., leaves, fruits) as well as the country of origin.

MY NOTES

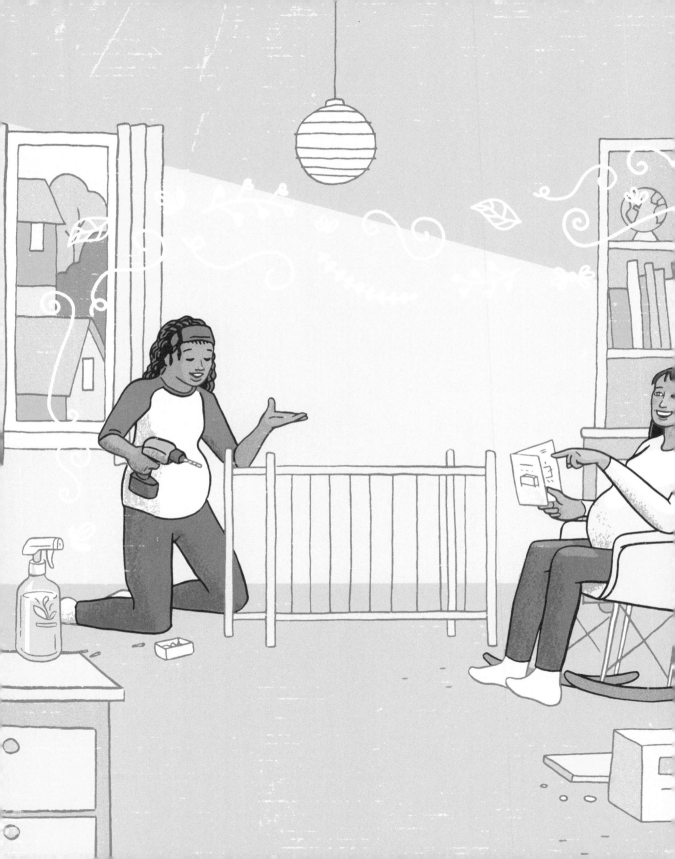

Chapter Two

AROMATHERAPY FOR PREGNANCY AND LABOR

The Benefits of Essential Oils for a Healthy Pregnancy

Pregnancy and labor are likely the most physically and emotionally complex and dynamic happenings of the human experience. Many honor these stages of a woman's life as rites of passage, defined by significant physical, emotional, and even spiritual metamorphosis. Everything is changing. Her body, her emotions, and her sense of self are all undergoing challenges, as perhaps are her intimate relationships and family dynamics. Although pregnancy and labor can involve the most incredible moments of a woman's life, the changes taking place are not necessarily easy to traverse. Indeed, rites of passage are by their very nature wrought with challenges to overcome. It is during these challenging times in our lives when aromatherapy can provide its most comforting support.

Wellness support from aromatherapy can assist the pregnant body in various ways. For example, essential oils are often called upon for digestive support through experiences of nausea and morning sickness, indigestion, and changes in bowel movements, such as constipation. As the body softens, stretches, and expands, there may be experiences of achy joints, muscle fatigue, and nerve pain. The skin sometimes needs support, as well. Some women experience hormonal acne; stretch marks on the abdomen, breasts, hips, or buttocks; and increased skin sensitivity. The circulatory system is also changing dramatically as it compensates for new blood vessels and increased blood volume. As the baby grows in size, pressure is placed on the return circulation from the legs and varicose veins and edema, or swelling, can occur. All of these physical changes during pregnancy can be supported with aromatherapy.

Aromatherapy is also an incredibly powerful and empowering tool to have on hand in the labor room, whether lending support to a tense birthing mother or providing a boost of encouragement. Essential oils can be very supportive allies after labor, too, as a woman's body heals and shifts to the demands of taking care of her newborn. There is a strong emotional component to pregnancy, labor, and the postpartum period, as well. Although there can be many moments of joy and excitement, changing hormone ecology, stress, fatigue, lack of sleep, and general worry can take an emotional toll. Supporting emotional well-being is where aromatherapy can really shine.

Pregnancy and Essential Oil Safety

For many women, pregnancy represents one of the strongest and most vital times of their lives. Growing a baby is no small task, and sometimes the overreaching message to pregnant women is a fearful one. Unfortunately, the same goes for essential oil safety and pregnancy.

There are a lot of conflicting opinions and mixed messages out there about which essential oils are safe to use, if any at all, and which methods of use pose the most risk.

One of the causes for confusion about essential oil safety and pregnancy is that there is little scientific information for or against it, which makes our decision-making processes more difficult to navigate. Most of the safety data we have is derived from animal research, the results of which do not easily translate to human use of essential oils. In this research, pregnant animals are exposed to doses of essential oils or essential oil components that are way beyond what one would experience with the external use of essential oils in aromatherapy practice. Nonetheless, it is the only safety information we have, and some believe that if an essential oil is deemed unsafe in animal research, we have to assume that it is unsafe during a human pregnancy.

There are four overarching safety concerns about using essential oils during pregnancy. These concerns include

1. The potential for essential oils to interfere with the health and normal development of the baby.

2. The possibility of essential oils negatively impacting the stability of the pregnancy, through either inducing a miscarriage or spontaneous abortion or causing preterm labor.

3. The possibility that essential oils could somehow interfere with reproductive hormones, either placing a woman's fertility or the stability of her pregnancy at risk or negatively impacting her ability to breastfeed.

4. The potential that the heightened skin sensitivity of a pregnant woman leads to increased opportunity for adverse skin reactions.

All four of these concerns are incredibly valid and must be addressed before any pregnant mother would feel assured about incorporating essential oils into her self-care practices.

In addressing the primary concern, that essential oils will interfere with the health and development of the baby, it is important to point out that at the time of this writing, there are no recorded instances of harm being caused to a growing fetus by essential oils used in massage and other external applications. Essential oils and essential oil components can cross the placental barrier, whereby they could theoretically be harmful to the health and development of the fetus. However, to reach the fetus, they must first be present at high enough levels in the mother's bloodstream. The recommended dilution of essential oils for aromatic and topical applications during pregnancy represents a very small dose. Furthermore, the amount of essential oil that is absorbed into the mother's bloodstream as a result of these external applications is even smaller. Therefore, through either aromatic or topical application, most essential oils pose very little risk of harming the health and development of the growing fetus when used externally at the recommended dose and dilution.

Regarding the second concern, addressing miscarriage or preterm labor, there are several essential oils that are said to have *emmenagogue* (stimulates uterine contractions) or *abortifacient* (causes spontaneous abortion) properties. However, according to many aromatherapy experts, these frightening and emotive words are not relevant when describing the external use of essential oils during a secure pregnancy. It is only when essential oils are ingested or used internally that the emmenagogue and abortifacient properties apply. In fact, there have been no adverse-event reports of miscarriage or spontaneous abortion as a result of the external use of essential oils. A small number of human case reports link two specific essential oils, pennyroyal and parsley seed, with miscarriage or death of a fetus. In these reported cases, these essential oils were taken internally at doses 100 and 200 times greater than the amounts used in "normal" aromatherapy applications. Nevertheless, the first trimester of a woman's pregnancy can be the most vulnerable, and if there is a history of miscarriage, most aromatherapists err on the side of caution and refrain from all essential oil use during this time. Similarly, although it is extremely unlikely that a secure pregnancy will be compromised with the topical or aromatic use of essential oils deemed emmenagogue, if a mother has previously had a miscarriage or gone into preterm labor, it would be prudent to avoid them.

Contrary to some claims, there is currently no evidence to substantiate that essential oils have enough influence over reproductive hormones to interfere with fertility, pregnancy, or breastfeeding when used externally. There is additional concern over exposing an infant to essential oils through breast milk. However, it is unlikely that more than 1 percent of an external dose of essential oil would end up in the breast milk via the mother's blood. This amount would be similar to the essential oils found in foods from the mother's diet that make it through to the breast milk. However, there is a possibility of exposing a nursing infant to essential oils if they are present in topical applications used on the breast prior to or between feedings, which is where the largest concern for exposure to the infant lies. If using essential oils topically on or around the breasts, it is best practice to apply them directly after feeding, not before, to allow for enough time for absorption and evaporation before contact with your baby's mouth.

Lastly, many women experience heightened skin sensitivity and photosensitivity during pregnancy, which can lead to an increased incidence of adverse skin reactions from the topical use of essential oils. Indeed, some essential oils, such as cinnamon, are generally considered contraindicated in pregnancy due to the increased potential of skin irritation rather than due to safety concerns for the baby or the pregnancy itself.

Aromatherapy has been used safely by pregnant mothers and their midwives, doulas, and nurses for decades. In fact, it appears that most essential oils are suitable for use during pregnancy when used appropriately; dose and dilution as well as internal versus external use are the major factors that influence the safety of an essential oil during pregnancy. Although it is not possible to say that the topical and aromatic use of essential oils during pregnancy and labor is 100 percent safe, it appears that the real danger to a baby and a pregnancy comes only with high doses, undiluted topical applications, and internal use. Nevertheless, below are lists of essential oils that, based on information from animal research, should not be used during pregnancy and breastfeeding and/or should be used only in moderation.

Pregnancy and Essential Oils

DO NOT USE	Aniseed • Araucaria • Bitter fennel • Black seed • Blue Cypress • Buchu • Calamint • Carrot seed • Cassia • Chaste tree (*Vitex*) • Cinnamon bark • Costus • Dill seed • Feverfew • Genipi • Hiba Wood • Ho leaf • Hyssop • Inula • Lantana • Mugwort • Mustard • Parsley seed • Pennyroyal • Rue • Sage, Dalmatian • Sage, Spanish • Sassafras • Savin • Spanish lavender • Star anise • Sweet birch • Sweet fennel • Tansy • Thuja • Western red cedar • Wintergreen • Wormwood • Yarrow
USE IN MODERATION	Bergamot • Champac • Cinnamon leaf • Clove • Cumin • Lemon basil • Lemon leaf • Lemon thyme • Lemon verbena • Lemongrass • May chang • Melissa • Myrtle • Oregano • Rosemary • Savory • Tea tree • Thyme
SAFE AT APPROPRIATE DOSES	Bay laurel • Benzoin • Black pepper • Cardamom • Clary sage • Coriander seed • Cypress • Eucalyptus • Frankincense • German chamomile • Ginger • Grapefruit • Helichrysum • Lavender • Lemon • Mandarin • Myrtle • Neroli • Palmarosa • Patchouli • Peppermint • Petitgrain • Roman chamomile • Rose geranium • Rose otto • Sweet basil • Sweet marjoram • Sweet orange • Vetiver • Ylang-ylang

The Three Trimesters

First Trimester

Breast tenderness, nausea, fatigue, and other symptoms of pregnancy begin in the first trimester. As hormones shift to maintain a pregnancy, emotions can swing. If you have a history of miscarriage, it is best to avoid essential oils during this time.

First Trimester Blends

Trying Not to Barf (Appetite Support) Personal Inhaler Blend

PREGNANCY, KIDS, ADULTS, SENIORS

TO MAKE THE BLEND

Add the essential oils to a small, dark glass dropper bottle and close tightly. Gently swirl to combine the oils. Label the bottle and store in a cool, dark place. Use it within 6 months of blending.

TO USE THE BLEND

Add 5 to 10 drops of oil to a personal aromatherapy inhaler wick. Be sure to label the inhaler. Alternatively, place 1 to 2 drops on a cotton ball or facial tissue to pull out and use as needed throughout the day.

TIP: Nausea is very personal, with different smells triggering different people. Each of these oils is appreciated for appetite support but might not come across that way to you. Before blending them together, try a gentle inhalation of each of these oils directly from the bottle to judge how it makes you feel. Then, with the bottles open, hold them together upright in your hands and gently circulate them under your nose to experience their combined aroma. If there is only one that you like, use that one!

AROMATIC

MAKES ½ OUNCE

1 teaspoon peppermint
  essential oil
1 teaspoon ginger
  essential oil
1 teaspoon lemon
  essential oil

I've Got This! Empowerment Roll-On

PREGNANCY, KIDS, ADULTS, SENIORS

1% DILUTION

TO MAKE THE BLEND

Add the essential oils to a roller bottle and gently swirl them together. Fill bottle to the top with the fractionated coconut oil. Close with the rollerball and cap and shake the bottle well. Label and store the blend in a cool, dark place. Use it within 6 months of blending.

TO USE THE BLEND

Gently dab the roller on the inner wrists, solar plexus, or heart chakra and/or behind your ears as needed when feeling overwhelmed.

AROMATIC, TOPICAL

MAKES ABOUT ½ OUNCE

1 drop bay laurel essential oil
1 drop vetiver essential oil
2 drops lavender essential oil
1 tablespoon fractionated coconut oil or calendula herbal-infused oil

Facial Glow Blend

PREGNANCY, TEENS, ADULTS, SENIORS

1% DILUTION

TO MAKE THE BLEND

Add the essential oils to a dark glass bottle with a pump or dropper, then add the hazelnut and jojoba oils. Close the bottle and shake vigorously. Label bottle, store in a cool, dark place, and use it within 6 months of blending.

TO USE THE BLEND

Apply a small amount to the palm of your hand, and using your fingers, gently massage the blend onto your face and upper back once or twice a day as part of a skin care routine.

TOPICAL

MAKES ABOUT 1 OUNCE

3 drops German chamomile essential oil
3 drops lavender essential oil
1 drop rose geranium essential oil
1 drop cedarwood essential oil
1 tablespoon cold-pressed hazelnut oil
1 tablespoon jojoba oil

Don't Touch Me! Breast Balm

PREGNANCY, TEENS, ADULTS

1% DILUTION

TO MAKE THE BLEND

Add the essential oils to a dark glass bottle with a pump or dropper, then add the calendula herbal-infused oil. Close the bottle and shake vigorously. Label the bottle, store in a cool, dark place, and use it within 6 months of blending. Double the recipe if needed.

TO USE THE BLEND

Use a small amount of balm to gently massage each breast for after-bath care. Use circular movements in the direction of the heart. Alternatively, mix 1 teaspoon into 1 cup Epsom salt, pour the mixture into the bath, and soak for at least 10 minutes with breasts submerged.

TOPICAL, PHOTOSENSITIZING

MAKES ABOUT 2 OUNCES

8 drops cypress essential oil

2 drops rosemary essential oil

3 drops grapefruit essential oil

3 drops frankincense essential oil

4 tablespoons calendula herbal-infused oil or other nut oil or olive oil

Second Trimester

Moving into the second trimester of pregnancy, you may find that clothes are no longer fitting. Stretch marks may begin to appear on the abdomen, hips, breasts, or buttocks. As the body starts softening, opening, and expanding, aches and pains become more common. Standing for long periods of time can become uncomfortable, and getting a good night's sleep may start proving more difficult.

Second Trimester Blends

Stretchy Skin Balm

PREGNANCY, TEENS, ADULTS, SENIORS   1% DILUTION

TO MAKE THE BALM

In a small glass bowl, combine the coconut oil, shea butter, and vitamin E oil, and stir vigorously until completely blended. If unable to blend, gently heat the coconut oil and shea butter on warm in the oven until liquid, allow to cool slightly, and add the vitamin E oil. After the base oils are thoroughly blended, add the essential oils, stir well, and scoop into a clean glass jar with a tight-fitting lid. Label the jar, store in a cool, dark place, and use it within 6 months of mixing.

TO USE THE BALM

For use from the fourth month of pregnancy and onward. Apply balm to the belly, hips, breasts, and buttocks once a day. You can also use it in small amounts locally on affected areas.

TOPICAL

MAKES ABOUT 1 CUP

½ cup unrefined coconut oil (solid at room temperature)

½ cup shea butter

20 drops vitamin E oil

25 drops frankincense essential oil

25 drops patchouli essential oil

7 drops helichrysum essential oil

5 drops rose otto essential oil or neroli essential oil

Deep Heat Massage Oil

1% DILUTION

TO MAKE THE MASSAGE OIL

Add the essential oils to a dark glass bottle with a pump or dropper, then add the olive oil. Close the bottle and shake it vigorously. Label and store the bottle in a cool, dark place, and use it within 6 months of blending.

TO USE THE MASSAGE OIL

Use massage oil as needed to support movement and relaxation of the muscles and joints. Great if used after yoga, stretching, or exercise. Be sure to wash hands after use.

TOPICAL

MAKES ABOUT 2 OUNCES

8 drops ginger essential oil

6 drops black pepper essential oil

2 drops rosemary essential oil

4 tablespoons cold-pressed olive oil

Sweet Dreams Pillow Spray

PREGNANCY, CHILDREN 6+, TEENS, ADULTS, SENIORS

1% DILUTION

TO MAKE THE SPRAY

Add the essential oils to a 2-ounce glass bottle with an aromatizer and swirl the oils until well blended. Fill the rest of the bottle with the distilled water, secure the lid, and shake it vigorously. Label the bottle, keep it stored away from the reach of children in a cool, dark place, and use it within 3 months of blending.

TO USE THE SPRAY

Shake the bottle vigorously before use. Spray 2 or 3 pumps on your pillow before bed. For dispersed coverage, make sure your pillow is at least 1 foot away. This spray may stain white pillowcases. Avoid spraying in the face and eyes.

AROMATIC

MAKES 2 OUNCES

3 drops clary sage essential oil

2 drops ylang-ylang essential oil

2 drops lavender essential oil

1 drop sweet marjoram essential oil

¼ cup distilled water

Third Trimester

By the time the third trimester comes around, increased weight and abdominal pressure from the growing baby can back up the bowels and slow circulation. Constipation, varicose veins, hemorrhoids, and swelling in the lower legs are common. There can also be a lot of excitement about the upcoming labor and, if it's your first pregnancy, perhaps a bit of anxiety, too.

Third Trimester Blends

Isn't That Swell? Circulation Support Blend

PREGNANCY, TEENS, ADULTS, SENIORS   1% DILUTION

TO MAKE THE BLEND

Add the essential oils to a dark glass bottle with a pump or dropper, then add the sesame oil. Close the bottle and shake vigorously. Label the bottle, store in a cool, dark place, and use it within 6 months of blending.

TO USE THE BLEND

Best used when lying down and feet are elevated above the level of the heart. Application is easiest when you can lie down and relax and have someone else help you out. Apply a small amount of the blend to your hands and gently massage your legs, starting with the feet and ankles and working up toward the knees, thighs, and groin. The direction of massage should always flow toward the heart.

TOPICAL, PHOTOSENSITIZING

MAKES 2 OUNCES

3 drops cypress essential oil
2 drops grapefruit essential oil
2 drops coriander essential oil
1 drop rosemary essential oil
¼ cup sesame oil or other vegetable or nut oil

TIP: Please note that this blend and course of action might be supportive when a mild case of swelling is present but not if preeclampsia is present. Be careful not to apply direct pressure on varicose veins.

A Bit Backed Up Bowel Belly Massage Blend

1% DILUTION

TO MAKE THE MASSAGE OIL

Add the essential oils to a dark glass bottle with a pump or dropper, then add the olive oil. Close the bottle and shake vigorously. Label the bottle, store in a cool, dark place, and use it within 6 months of blending.

TO USE THE MASSAGE OIL

Lie flat on your back if comfortable, or if not, lie on your left side. Apply a small amount of the massage oil to the palm of your hand and gently spread around the belly starting on the lower right side of the abdomen and moving up the right side, across to the left side, and then down the left side. Repeat with varying levels of comfortable pressure for 5 to 10 minutes as needed.

TOPICAL, PHOTOSENSITIZING

MAKES 2 OUNCES

3 drops ginger essential oil

3 drops cardamom essential oil

2 drops lemon essential oil

¼ cup cold-pressed olive oil or other nut or vegetable oil

Inflamed in the Veins Vascular Support Gel

PREGNANCY, TEENS, ADULTS, SENIORS   1% DILUTION

TO MAKE THE GEL

In a glass bowl, combine the aloe vera gel and the essential oils and stir together thoroughly. Transfer the mixture to a glass jar with a tight-fitting lid. Label the jar, store in a cool, dark place, and use it within 1 month of blending.

TO USE THE GEL

Gently dab small amounts of gel on swollen or sore veins and hemorrhoids as needed, up to three times a day.

TOPICAL

MAKES ABOUT ½ CUP

½ cup aloe vera gel

10 drops lavender essential oil

10 drops rose geranium essential oil

7 drops Roman chamomile essential oil

5 drops white pine essential oil or spruce essential oil

Pregnancy and Postpartum Concerns

Miscarriage and Preterm Birth

There is nothing simple about the emotional or physical experience of losing a child to miscarriage. Even a premature birth to an otherwise healthy baby can be incredibly grievous and stressful. Emotional support is of paramount importance during these times, and aromatherapy really shines here. These blends do well as personal inhalers and in aromatherapy jewelry, diffusion blends, and personal aromatherapy mists. They are most effective in conjunction with other forms of care, including talk therapy, yoga, and meditation.

Blends for Miscarriage and Preterm Birth

Blend for Grief Support

CHILDREN 6+, TEENS, ADULTS, SENIORS

TO MAKE THE BLEND

Add the essential oils to a small, dark glass dropper bottle and swirl the oils to mix. Cap the bottle tightly and make sure to label the blend. Store the bottle in a cool, dark place, and use it within 6 months of blending.

TO USE THE BLEND

Apply 10 to 15 drops to the wick of an aromatherapy inhaler and use as needed. Similarly, you can apply 1 or 2 drops to aromatherapy jewelry, a cotton ball, or a facial tissue to carry with you to use as needed. Or you can add 15 to 30 drops to 1 ounce of distilled water to use as an aromatherapy mist. If using an aromatherapy diffuser, follow the manufacturer's instructions regarding the number of essential oil drops to use per diffusion. Diffuse for 30 minutes at a time one or two times a day.

AROMATIC

MAKES ½ OUNCE

1½ teaspoons rosemary essential oil

1½ teaspoons vetiver essential oil

Blend for Anger Support

TO MAKE THE BLEND

Add the essential oils to a small, dark glass dropper bottle and swirl the oils to mix. Cap the bottle tightly and make sure to label the blend. Store it in a cool, dark place, and use it within 6 months of blending.

TO USE THE BLEND

Apply 10 to 15 drops to the wick of an aromatherapy inhaler; 1 or 2 drops to aromatherapy jewelry, a cotton ball, or a facial tissue; or 15 to 30 drops to 1 ounce of distilled water to use as an aromatherapy mist. If using an aromatherapy diffuser, follow the manufacturer's instructions regarding the number of essential oil drops to use per diffusion. Diffuse for 30 minutes one or two times a day.

AROMATIC

MAKES ½ OUNCE

1 teaspoon lemon essential oil

1 teaspoon sweet basil essential oil

½ teaspoon oregano essential oil

½ teaspoon black pepper essential oil

Blend for Sadness Support

TO MAKE THE BLEND

Add the essential oils to a small, dark glass dropper bottle and swirl the oils to mix. Cap the bottle tightly and make sure to label the blend. Store it in a cool, dark place, and use it within 6 months of blending.

TO USE THE BLEND

Apply 10 to 15 drops to the wick of an aromatherapy inhaler; 1 or 2 drops to aromatherapy jewelry, a cotton ball, or a facial tissue; or 15 to 30 drops to 1 ounce of distilled water to use as an aromatherapy mist. If using an aromatherapy diffuser, follow the manufacturer's instructions regarding the number of essential oil drops to use per diffusion. Diffuse for 30 minutes one or two times a day.

AROMATIC

MAKES ABOUT ½ OUNCE

1 teaspoon sweet marjoram essential oil

1 teaspoon sweet orange essential oil

1 teaspoon rose geranium essential oil

10 drops rose otto essential oil

Postpartum

The weeks and months following labor are alive with changes for both you and the baby. Aromatherapy can offer healing support through experiences such as after pains, wound healing, and cracked nipples or sore breasts. As hormones shift yet again, the baby blues can set in, as can fatigue and irritability from sleeplessness and feeling overwhelmed.

Blends for Postpartum

Not My Nipples! Soothing Salve

PREGNANCY, BREASTFEEDING   0.25% DILUTION

TO MAKE THE SALVE

In a stainless steel saucepan, combine the lanolin and cocoa butter, and gently heat on low until the butters are melted and liquid. Set aside to cool. In a small glass bowl, add the calendula herbal-infused oil and blend the essential oils into it, mixing well. Once the lanolin and cocoa butter mixture has cooled, slowly add the herbal and essential oil blend while stirring. Once blended, pour into clean salve tins or jars to set. Label the tins, store in a cool, dark place, and use it within 6 months of blending.

TO USE THE SALVE

Apply as needed to nipples. Apply only immediately after feeding, not before. Leave plenty of time for absorption and evaporation, leaving no salve to come in direct contact with your baby's mouth during feeding time.

TOPICAL

MAKES ABOUT 1 CUP

¼ cup lanolin or shea butter
½ cup cocoa butter
¼ cup calendula
   herbal-infused oil
10 drops lavender
   essential oil
10 drops German chamomile
   essential oil

Deeply Rooted Calm Diffusion Blend

POSTPARTUM, CHILDREN 6+, TEENS, ADULTS, SENIORS

TO MAKE THE BLEND

Add the essential oils to a dark glass dropper bottle and swirl the oils to mix. Label the blend, store it in a cool, dark place, and use it within 6 months of blending.

TO USE THE BLEND

Apply 10 to 15 drops to the wick of an aromatherapy inhaler and use as needed. Similarly, you can apply 1 or 2 drops to aromatherapy jewelry, a cotton ball, or a facial tissue to carry with you to use as needed. Or add 15 to 30 drops to 1 ounce of distilled water to use as an aromatherapy mist. If using an aromatherapy diffuser, follow the manufacturer's instructions regarding the number of essential oil drops to use per diffusion. Diffuse for 10 to 15 minutes at a time one or two times a day.

AROMATIC

MAKES ABOUT ½ OUNCE

- 1 teaspoon frankincense essential oil
- 1 teaspoon sweet marjoram essential oil
- ½ teaspoon clary sage essential oil
- ½ teaspoon vetiver or patchouli essential oil

Wound and Trauma Aftercare Support Sitz Bath

POSTPARTUM

1% DILUTION

TO MAKE THE SITZ BATH

Combine all of the essential oils with the herbal-infused oil in a glass measuring cup and stir well. Add the Epsom salt, mix thoroughly, and transfer the mixture to a glass jar with a tight-fitting lid. Label the jar, store in a cool, dark place, and use it within 6 months of blending.

TO USE THE SITZ BATH

Add ⅓ cup to comfortably warm bathwater, enough to submerge the genitals. Soak for 10 to 15 minutes, making sure that wounds stay clean. Makes enough for two or three sitz baths.

TOPICAL

MAKES ABOUT 1 CUP

- 2 drops lavender essential oil
- 2 drops German chamomile essential oil
- 2 drops rosemary essential oil
- 2 drops helichrysum essential oil
- ¼ cup St. John's wort herbal-infused oil
- ¾ cup Epsom salt

SAFETY TIPS

✦ Essential oils should not be used in a birth pool because after delivery, a baby may surface with his or her eyes open.

✦ Do not use essential oils during the first trimester if there is a history of miscarriage. Consider avoiding essential oil use all together if there is a history of miscarriage or preterm labor.

✦ Increased photosensitivity and general skin sensitivity are possible during pregnancy. You may find that essential oils that you have used in the past without reaction are now the cause of minor to major irritation. If unsure, you can always resort to a patch test. Avoid direct sun exposure after using essential oils with known phototoxicity. You may be particularly vulnerable to photosensitizing reactions during your pregnancy.

✦ Inhalation poses the fewest safety concerns. One drop on a pillowcase or cotton ball or in a diffuser is sometimes all that is needed.

✦ Minimize daily use. It is best to use essential oils only when you really need them.

BEST PRACTICES

✦ Keep your pregnancy and birth care team informed about your aromatherapy practices, and seek the advice of a qualified health practitioner if you are uncertain whether essential oils are safe for you and your baby.

✦ Always label your blends and aromatherapy products with all essential oils and other ingredients. It is also helpful to put the dilution on the label as well as indicate for whom in your home it is safe to use.

✦ Keep blends and aromatherapy products stored away from heat and light and out
of the reach of children or pets.

MY NOTES

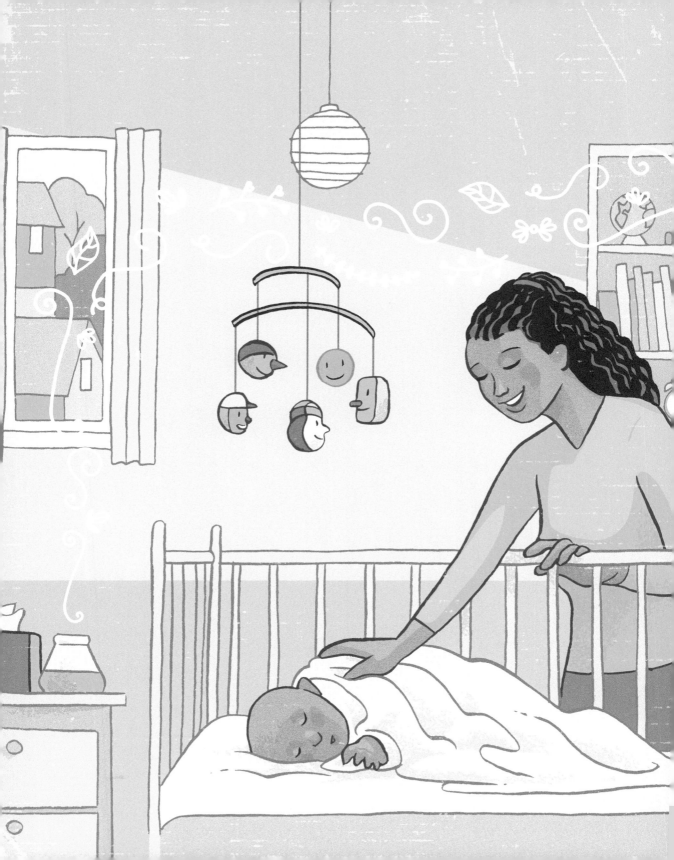

Chapter Three

BLENDS FOR BABIES

Babies and Essential Oil Safety

When delving into aromatherapy, many parents want to know about how to use essential oils safely with their newborn babies and infants. This is a highly debated topic among aromatherapists and essential oil safety experts, and for good reason. Being new to a world full of sights, smells, sounds, and sensations comes with a gentle sensitivity that can be easily overwhelmed even by natural substances, like essential oils. In light of this, special safety concerns must be addressed in regard to aromatherapy on or around your baby. However, when approached safely, aromatherapy can be an incredibly fun, interactive, and supportive tool for both you and your young one.

Babies and Special Safety Concerns

There is nothing quite like the smell of a newborn baby. It is an aroma that is difficult to describe yet instills such deep sensations of love and protection. By the time a baby is born, they are already familiar with how you smell, too, and as their eyesight develops, they will rely on both the sound of your voice and your innate scent for recognition and bonding. In fact, many experts say that smelling like yourself, devoid of aromas that cover up your natural scent, is best for establishing a connection and getting to know one another over these first few months of life.

Although a baby's senses of hearing and smell are fully developed at birth, their skin is not. During the first 12 weeks of life, your newborn's skin undergoes significant changes that leave it more vulnerable to damage and adverse reactions to essential oils. It is also much thinner and more permeable than your own. In addition, your newborn's internal organs are not fully developed and are less able to efficiently process essential oil components that may absorb through the skin. In simple terms, your newborn is not yet equipped to process or protect against chemicals that they are exposed to, including essential oils. This vulnerability is even more pronounced with preterm infants.

Most aromatherapy and essential oil safety experts agree that parents should refrain from using essential oils on or around infants younger than three months of age, including both topical and aromatic use. If your baby is preterm, the additional precaution of waiting until three months after the intended due date is considered best practice. Lastly, it can be helpful to remember that during these first three months of life, your baby does not need essential oils to be well—love, tenderness, touch, food, and sleep are the most important things.

How Young Is Too Young?

By the time your baby is three months old, they are able to see your face more clearly. Perhaps they are full of smiles and facial expressions and carry on babbling conversations, mimicking your every sound. By this time, they are strong enough to support their own head, open and close their hands, shake toys, and swat at dangling objects. They will also be able to put their hands in their mouth and will be grabbing for anything they can reach, including opened bottles of essential oils.

You may have been noticing changes in your baby's skin, such as baby acne, milia, and cradle cap. Perhaps your baby has encountered some digestive struggles with gas or constipation. Your baby could also be struggling with colic; the intense inconsolable crying, restlessness, and fussiness are incredibly stressful and can take an emotional toll on you both. It is during these times when we desperately want to provide the best for our babies and support them through their discomforts in the most natural way possible. Aromatherapy can be wonderfully soothing for both baby and parents, but safety should always come first.

There is a bit of debate about whether or not it is safe to use essential oils topically during this stage or if the use of essential oils should be limited to aromatic use only. Your baby's skin is still maturing at this age, so topical use of essential oils should be restricted to mild, non-irritating, non-photosensitizing oils that have been diluted to no more than 0.25 percent. This amount equates to 1 drop of essential oil per ounce of carrier oil. It is also recommended that you perform a patch test at this dilution prior to applying any essential oil to the skin via massage.

Sometimes massage with unscented oil and loving touch are all you need to soothe your baby. However, if choosing to include essential oils into your massage blends, be sure to not apply to areas that could end up in your baby's mouth or up your baby's nose, such as the lower arms, wrists and hands, feet, fingers, or toes. In addition, it is of paramount importance to ensure that massage blends that contain essential oils are not applied to or near your baby's face.

If choosing to diffuse essential oils around your three- to six-month-old, placing 1 or 2 drops in a diffuser and diffusing for 5 minutes at a time no more than three times a day is all that is recommended. During this time, you should make sure that the space is well ventilated, and keep an eye out for signs of discomfort, such as eye irritation and/or crying.

It is generally considered best practice to introduce babies to one essential oil at a time, rather than using a blend. This introduction can be achieved by wearing it diluted on your own skin first so that your baby can get used to the smell, and you can watch for signs of sensitivities or dislikes before using it topically or aromatically with them. Be sure to use the same dilution on yourself as you would on your baby, and apply it only to areas that will not come in direct contact with their mouth.

General Safety Precautions for Babies 6 to 24 Months

The period of 6 to 24 months is marked by rapid growth and development of your little one. Teething begins and, by 24 months, your infant is well on the way to sprouting a full set of baby teeth. Babies quickly evolve from rolling onto their bellies to scooting and crawling, and finally taking their first steps. Babbling sounds turn into heartwarming words and intelligible phrases. You begin to notice infants learning to express themselves and developing their own personalities.

Common colds and upper-respiratory congestion are common during this period, especially when your baby is exposed to other children. By now you have likely learned to battle with diaper rash and are seeking workarounds for the peak in separation anxiety that comes with going back to work or dropping off your child at day care. Hopefully you have found a good nighttime routine, one that works for you both, and are having only occasional trouble getting your baby to sleep or waking in the night to soothe bad dreams.

Remember with topical application to avoid the face and any parts of the body that could end up in the baby's mouth, including lower arms, hands, and feet. Focus on the chest, abdomen, and upper legs instead. Follow your dilutions carefully; the amount of essential oil per ounce of carrier oil deemed safe for a 24-month-old will be more than what is considered safe for a 6-month-old.

Since babies love to splash and play, some aromatherapy experts advise not using essential oils in the bath in order to avoid contact with the mouth, eyes, or other sensitive membranes. However, if you want to use essential oils in the bath, they must be diluted in a carrier oil or liquid castile soap first in order to avoid coming in direct, undiluted contact with your baby's sensitive skin. Also, pay close attention so that your baby doesn't swallow the bathwater.

If using essential oils aromatically, it is advised that you altogether avoid direct inhalation, including exposing your baby to strong essential oil vapors straight from the bottle and the use of cotton balls or personal inhalers that could be inadvertently placed in their mouth. It is also unsafe to place essential oils or aromatherapy preparations of any kind into your baby's nose.

Diffusing essential oils is considered to be the safest aromatic method of use around babies. However, as your baby won't be able to get away from strong smells, it is important that you diffuse only essential oils that are deemed safe for use at this stage of life and that you pay attention for signs of distress, such as crying, fussiness, and rubbing of irritated, watery eyes. It is also advised that you limit exposure to only a few minutes a day a few times a day, being sure to take breaks, and avoid overexposure through frequent use.

Hydrosols: A Safe Aromatherapy Alternative to Essential Oils

Essential oils are not the only tools in the aromatherapy tool set. Providing an incredibly safe alternative to essential oils are hydrosols, also known as hydrolats, which are water-based extracts that are a by-product of essential oil production. During the steam distillation of essential oils, water that has evaporated through the plant material and captured the essential oil molecules is condensed and separated. These water-based extracts carry with them many of the water-soluble therapeutic compounds of the mother plant material as well as highly diluted compounds from the essential oil.

Hydrosols are very different in nature than essential oils, both chemically and therapeutically. They provide a gentle, safe, yet effective alternative to essential oils, especially for the very young or other sensitive populations. In fact, high-quality hydrosols that are free from preservatives or synthetic ingredients are so mild in their activity that some sources consider them safe even for use on or around infants from zero to three months. Hydrosols can be spritzed around a room, misted onto bedclothes, enjoyed in the bath, or in some cases, used in compresses directly on delicate, troubled skin.

Make sure when you are purchasing hydrosols that you read the label carefully and avoid those that contain anything other than just the hydrosol. For example, because hydrosols have a limited shelf life, many aromatherapy retailers will add alcohol for preservation and shelf stability. Added ingredients can make hydrosols irritating to delicate baby skin. Also note that "prepared waters" or "aromatic waters" may not be true hydrosols and therefore are not unequivocally safe for use. It is important that the label indicates the hydrosol was produced from stream distillation and does not contain any added ingredients. Keep hydrosols in your refrigerator in clean, sterile containers, and use them within three to six months of opening. Discard if cloudiness, mold, or unpleasant smells develop.

SUPPORTS	HYDROSOL / HYDROLAT
Irritated, inflamed skin	Chamomile, rose, lavender, calendula, melissa
Restfulness and sleep	Chamomile, rose, lavender, melissa, clary sage
Calm and settled digestion	Chamomile, lavender, melissa
Breathing through nose and mouth	Frankincense, lavender

Application Guidelines for Three to Six Months

Some aromatherapy and essential oil safety experts suggest that essential oils not be used topically for this age group. Other experts suggest that a 0.25 percent dilution (1 drop per ounce) is safe for topical use for this age group. Perform a patch test at this dilution before applying to large areas of the body. Make sure to avoid contact with the baby's face and any parts of their body that could end up in their mouth.

When diffusing essential oils around this age group, make sure that you are using only 1 or 2 drops in your diffuser. Diffuse for 5 minutes at a time for a maximum of three times a day, and avoid diffusing every day. Make sure the room is well ventilated, and keep a close eye on your little one for signs of irritation.

SAFE AND USEFUL ESSENTIAL OILS FOR BABIES THREE TO SIX MONTHS

* Dill weed
* German chamomile
* Lavender
* Roman chamomile
* Sweet orange

Blends for Three to Six Months

Baby Powder Blend

BABIES 3+ MONTHS

TO MAKE THE POWDER

In a spice or coffee grinder, grind the calendula flowers into a fine powder. Sift the ground flowers and remove any unground pieces. Combine 1 tablespoon of the powder with the kaolin clay and arrowroot in a glass measuring cup. Add the essential oils (if using) and continue stirring until the oil is evenly mixed into the powder and there are no clumps. Scoop into a glass jar, one with a perforated lid if available (clean spice jars work well). Label and store the powder in a cool, dark place, and use it within 6 months of blending.

TO USE THE POWDER

Use daily as you would regular baby powder, applying to clean, dry skin. Stop using if skin irritation appears or gets worse.

TOPICAL

MAKES ABOUT 1 CUP

1½ to 2 tablespoons dried calendula or rose flowers

¾ cup kaolin clay

1 to 2 tablespoons arrowroot power

2 drops lavender essential oil (optional)

2 drops German chamomile essential oil (optional)

Soothe My Skin Rinse

PREGNANCY, BABIES 3+ MONTHS, CHILDREN 2+, SENIORS

TO MAKE THE RINSE

Pour the distilled water into a glass measuring cup. Place the measuring cup in a pan and fill the pan with water until it reaches halfway up the side of the cup. Gently heat until the distilled water is slightly warmer than room temperature. Once warmed, remove from heat and add the hydrosol of your choosing. Pour the rinse into a glass jar with a tight-fitting lid. Refrigerate and use the blend within 24 hours. Stir well before use. It is safe to use this rinse once daily through the duration of need.

TO USE THE RINSE

Add all of the rinse directly to bathwater if you want to soak. It can also be used as a final rinse to the scalp after shampooing. Make sure all soap is thoroughly rinsed away, and gently pour the rinse from the measuring cup over the scalp. This rinse can also be used in a compress or to dampen wiping cloths when changing diapers. Submerge a cloth or cotton pad and wring out completely before gently holding it to skin or dabbing skin. You can also place the rinse in a misting bottle and mist the skin (avoiding the face), then dry with a soft towel before applying massage oil or moisturizer.

TOPICAL

MAKES 1 CUP

½ cup distilled water
½ cup lavender hydrosol, German chamomile hydrosol, or rose hydrosol

TIP: Use rose hydrosol if there is dry skin present, lavender if redness present, and chamomile if milia or baby acne present.

Settled and Sleepy Diffusion or Room Mist Blend

PREGNANCY, BABIES 3+ MONTHS, CHILDREN 2+, TEENS, ADULTS, SENIORS

0.25% DILUTION

TO MAKE THE BLEND

Add the essential oil to a dark glass bottle with a cap or an aromatizer, then add clary sage hydrosol. Cap the bottle tightly, label, and store the blend in the refrigerator for up to 3 months.

TO USE THE BLEND

Shake vigorously before use. Fill an aromatherapy diffuser as indicated by the manufacturer. Diffuse for 5 minutes before putting your baby to bed. If needed throughout the night, diffuse once or twice more for a maximum of 5 minutes, making sure the door is open and the room well ventilated. An alternative to diffusion is using an aromatizer. Spritz several times around the room 5 to 10 minutes before putting your baby to bed. Do not spritz on or around your baby.

AROMATIC

MAKES 2 OUNCES

2 drops lavender essential oil or sweet orange essential oil
¼ cup clary sage hydrosol

TIP: If you or your baby don't like the scent of clary sage hydrosol, try chamomile, lavender, melissa, or frankincense hydrosol instead.

Blessed Belly Massage Blend

PREGNANCY, BABIES 3+ MONTHS, CHILDREN 2+, SENIORS

0.25% DILUTION

TO MAKE THE BLEND

Add the essential oil to a dark glass bottle with a pump or dropper, and then add the grapeseed oil. Close tightly and shake well to mix. Label and store the blend in a cool, dark, place, and use it within 6 months of blending.

TO USE THE BLEND

Shake the bottle vigorously before use. Warm a small amount of the blend in your hands and gently apply it to your baby's belly in a clockwise direction. You can also apply it to other areas, but avoid the lower arms, hands, and feet. Never apply the blend to your baby's face.

TOPICAL

MAKES 2 OUNCES

2 drops sweet orange essential oil, German chamomile essential oil, or dill weed essential oil
¼ cup grapeseed oil or cold-pressed olive oil

Application Guidelines for 6 to 24 Months

Aromatherapy and essential oil safety experts suggest a maximum 0.5 percent dilution (2 drops per ounce) for topical use on babies 6 to 24 months old. Perform a patch test at this dilution before applying to large areas of the body. Make sure to avoid contact with the face and any parts of the body that could end up in your baby's mouth.

When diffusing essential oils around this age group, make sure that you are using only 1 or 2 drops in your diffuser. Diffuse for 5 minutes at a time for a maximum of three times a day, and avoid diffusing every day. Make sure the room is well ventilated, and keep a close eye on your little one for signs of irritation.

SAFE AND USEFUL ESSENTIAL OILS FOR BABIES 6 TO 24 MONTHS

- Bergamot (bergapten-free)
- Cedarwood
- Fir needle
- Grapefruit
- Lemon
- Mandarin
- Neroli
- Patchouli
- Ravensara
- Rose geranium
- Rose otto
- Spruce
- Sweet marjoram
- Tangerine
- Tea tree
- White pine

Blends for 6 to 24 Months

Smooth Scalp Shampoo

BABIES 6+ MONTHS, CHILDREN 2+, SENIORS

0.5% DILUTION

TO MAKE THE SHAMPOO

Combine the shampoo and olive oil in a glass measuring cup. Stir until thoroughly mixed. Add the essential oils and continue stirring until all ingredients are mixed together well. Pour the mixture into a glass or polyethylene terephthalate (PET)–free plastic bottle with a pump. Label and store the shampoo in a cool, dark place, and use it within 6 months of blending.

TO USE THE SHAMPOO

During bath time, squirt half a pump or less into the palm of your hand. Using your fingertips, gently apply to your baby's scalp and massage the scalp for several minutes before rinsing. Be careful to not allow any shampoo to drip on or near your baby's eyes or face. Be prepared for separation of ingredients in the bottle, always shaking well before use.

TIP: For a thicker shampoo with added moisture, use olive oil. For a thinner shampoo, use lavender hydrosol, but be prepared for separation of ingredients in the bottle. Use a clear glass bottle or PET-free clear plastic bottle so you can keep an eye out for separation of ingredients.

TOPICAL

MAKES 2 OUNCES

3 tablespoons unscented shampoo or liquid castile soap

1 tablespoon cold-pressed olive oil or lavender hydrosol

2 drops patchouli essential oil

2 drops cedarwood or lavender essential oil

Breathe Easy Chest Rub

0.5% DILUTION

TO MAKE THE RUB

Gently warm the coconut oil in a double boiler or bain-marie until it is soft enough to stir. Remove the coconut oil from heat and allow it to cool until it's just warmer than body temperature (or it's just beginning to solidify). It should be close to room temperature when adding essential oils. Add the essential oils and stir well until thoroughly blended. Scoop the blend into a glass jar with a tight-fitting lid, and label clearly. Store in a cool, dark place, and use it within 6 to 12 months of blending.

TO USE THE RUB

Dip a clean index finger into the jar and scoop out a pea-sized dollop of the rub. Place the dollop in the palm of your hand and rub your hands together until they are warm and the rub is melted and evenly dispersed over your palms. With gentle, upward stroking motions, apply the rub to your baby's chest, upper arms, and upper back. Avoid the lower arms, hands, feet, and other body parts that could end up in your baby's mouth. Do not apply on or near your baby's face. Apply two or three times a day as needed to support breathing.

TOPICAL

MAKES ½ CUP

- ½ cup unrefined coconut oil (solid at room temperature)
- 8 drops sweet marjoram essential oil or tea tree essential oil
- 8 drops white pine essential oil

"Console Me" Loving Touch Massage Blend

BABIES 6+ MONTHS, CHILDREN 2+, SENIORS

0.5% DILUTION

TO MAKE THE BLEND

Add the essential oils to a dark glass bottle with a pump or dropper, and then add the olive oil. Close the bottle tightly, shake well, and be sure to label the blend. Store in a cool, dark place, and use it within 6 months of blending.

TO USE THE BLEND

Shake the bottle vigorously before use. Apply a small amount to your hands and rub them together to warm them. Using gentle, rhythmic motions, apply the blend to your baby's belly, flowing in a clockwise direction. You can also apply it to the upper arms, legs, and chest, but avoid the lower arms, hands, and feet. Never apply the blend to your baby's face.

TOPICAL

MAKES 2 OUNCES

2 drops sweet orange
  essential oil
2 drops rose otto essential oil
¼ cup cold-pressed olive oil or
  coconut oil

SAFETY TIPS

- Do not use essential oils on or around babies younger than three months old.

- Do not allow babies to ingest essential oils, and keep all aromatherapy products away from the reach of your young ones.

- Avoid using essential oils in the bath. Use hydrosols instead.

- Make sure to follow dilution ratios carefully, and never apply essential oils undiluted to your baby's skin.

- When applying essential oils topically, avoid applying them to body parts that could inadvertently end up in your baby's mouth or nose, such as hands, lower arms, wrists, and feet. Do not apply essential oils to your baby's face or up your baby's nose. Avoid all contact with the eyes, nose, and mouth.

- Do not use essential oils in the ears.

- Avoid using essential oils to clean toys that your baby puts in their mouth.

- Use only essential oils deemed safe for your baby's age group. Avoid essential oils that are known irritants and photosensitizers.

BEST PRACTICES

- Always speak to your pediatrician or other qualified health professional before using essential oils on or around your baby. Remember that not all difficulties can be supported with aromatherapy.

- Always use high-quality, 100-percent pure, organic (if possible) essential oils from reputable sources.

- If breastfeeding and using essential oils in your self-care regimen, be sure to wash your breasts and nipples thoroughly before feeding, or wait to apply said measures until after feeding, when there is plenty of time for absorption and evaporation. If you are having trouble with breastfeeding, try removing essential oils from all topical applications you might be using.

- Introduce babies to one essential oil at a time by wearing it on your skin at the dilution appropriate for their age group. Perform a patch test before applying to large areas of their skin.

- When diffusing essential oils, if your baby shows any signs of discomfort, such as eye irritation or crying, stop diffusing the oil and try again after some time. If your baby shows signs of irritation the second time, then stop the diffusion, and refrain from using that essential oil.

- Avoid exposing your baby's skin to direct sunlight immediately after using aromatherapy blends containing essential oils.

- Take breaks. There may be little need for daily use of essential oils. If you find you are exposing your baby to daily doses of essential oils, be sure to take at least a one-week break for every two weeks of use.

MY NOTES

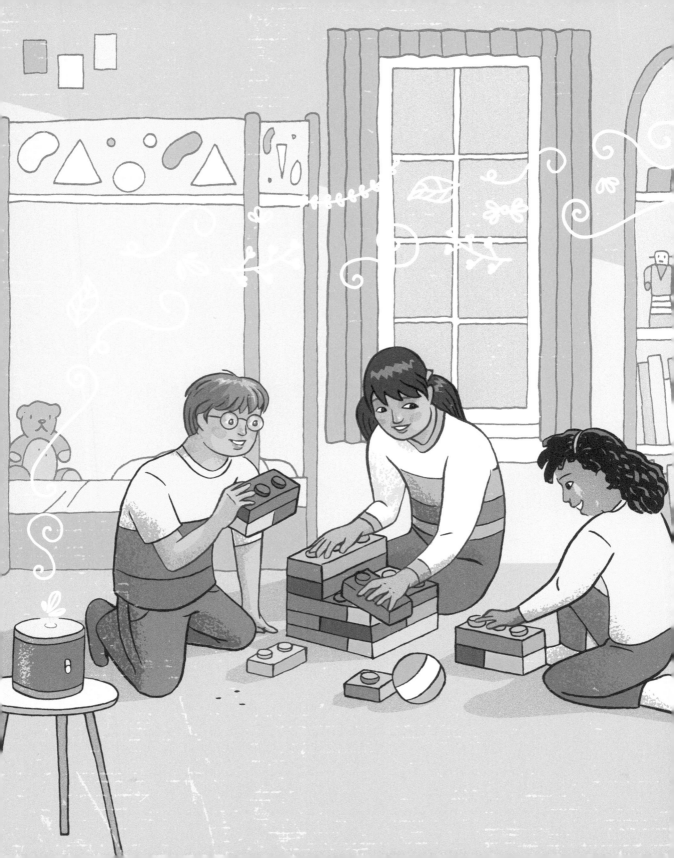

Chapter Four

AROMATHERAPY FOR KIDS

Benefits of Essential Oils for Children

As our babies grow up, challenges to their well-being become more diverse and complex. From ages 2 to 18, their bodies are rapidly growing and changing, demanding both more nutrition and more sleep. By the time they are six years old, their immune systems are fully mature, and you will have no doubt experienced more colds, flus, and tummy bugs than you ever thought possible. They explore the world with the verve of wildlings, as evidenced by their collection of bumps, bruises, and insect bites.

By the time our children reach high school, their impressions of the world are also rapidly changing. They are learning about self-expression, connection, friendships, and social norms (whether they like them or not) as they continue to explore their identity and sense of self. By now, your children's challenges to well-being may be more obvious and clearly defined: Dietary and airborne allergies, asthma, eczema, or digestive problems may have become the norm. They may also be struggling with restlessness at school, difficulty concentrating, or acting out in the classroom. Perhaps getting them to sit still and focus on their homework is becoming increasingly challenging.

With puberty, changes occur to body weight and shape, skin, body odor, voice, and hair. Moreover, just as our teenagers are reaching the peak of their physiological transition from childhood to adulthood, they are grappling with strong desires to fit in, to feel accepted, and to be independent from us. It is an emotionally charged epoch in your family's story, characterized by full-belly laughter, shouting matches, and slamming doors. Struggles with stress, anxiety, and depression are more common, as are issues surrounding your teens' developing adulthood; instead of returning with bumps and bruises, they now come home with confusion, hurt feelings, and broken hearts. Days off from school due to menstrual cramps, athletic injuries, respiratory infections, fatigue, or allergy flare-ups are likely commonplace.

Age 2 to age 18 is a huge expanse of time characterized by all the joys and troubles of growing up human in this world. There is so much that aromatherapy can do to sup-port your children as they journey through toddlerhood into adulthood and traverse the various physical and emotional challenges that characterize these different eras of their young lives. As your child's needs grow and change, so will both the wellness benefits and safety protocols of essential oil use. In fact, each stage, from toddler to teen, comes with its own essential oil safety guidelines and precautions. Generally speaking, the older your child gets, the less restrictions are placed on which essential oils and which dilutions are deemed safe. However, your aromatherapy choices will remain dependent upon your well-ness goals and what you are hoping to achieve through the use of essential oils.

Essential Oils to Avoid at All Ages

TOXIC	Ajowan • Bitter almond • Boldo • Buchu • Calamus • Camphor, brown and yellow • Horseradish • Mustard • Rue • Sassafras • Savin • Tansy • Thuja • Wormseed • Wormwood
POTENTIALLY HAZARDOUS	Bitter fennel • Cassia • Garlic • Hyssop • Mugwort • Onion • Pennyroyal • Santolina • Savory • Spanish lavender • Sweet birch • Wintergreen

Essential Oil Safety and Application Guidelines for Children Ages 2 to 6

It is important to remember that the immune systems of children in this age group are not yet fully developed, and they will still be sensitive to aromatic and topical applications of essential oils. Overuse of essential oils or applying essential oils that have not been properly diluted could lead to adverse skin reactions more quickly and easily for this age group. These types of reactions usually appear directly after essential oil use and manifest as irritation, itching, blistering, redness, or phototoxicity (being very easily sunburned). These types of reactions could also indicate an allergy, so it is important to patch-test essential oils at the appropriate dilution before applying them to large areas of the body.

In addition, it is believed that sensitization reactions to essential oils are more likely to develop for this age group than for older children and adults. These types of reactions are characterized by an essential oil becoming intolerable to your child's skin and/or immune system over a period of time and are caused by overexposure to the same essential oil, including those properly diluted, and by excessive use of essential oils in general. Sensitization reactions are usually delayed reactions that behave like an allergy, and in some cases, the sensitivity never goes away.

When using essential oils topically, you can avoid both adverse skin reactions and sensitization by making sure to dilute essential oils properly and by avoiding overuse and daily exposure. One percent dilution for topical application of essential oils is considered standard for this age group. This amount equates to 9 drops per 1 ounce of carrier or base. Similar to the application guidelines with babies, be sure not to apply essential oils to areas of the body that could end up in your child's mouth or eyes. In addition, even diluted essential oils should never be applied on or near your child's face and certainly never placed inside your child's nose. Essential oils can be used safely in the bath, but the same safety precautions still apply as for younger children and babies: dilute, dilute, dilute, and avoid contact with the mouth, eyes, or other sensitive membranes.

Aromatic use of essential oils should be limited to diffusion using half the amount of essential oil recommended for your diffuser and for a maximum of 30 minutes at a time, no more than three times a day. It is always best practice to take breaks and refrain from using essential oils every day. Direct inhalation from essential oil bottles, cotton balls, and personal inhalers is not recommended, especially if the child is unsupervised. Most poisoning and toxicity reactions that have been reported for children in this age group were a result of accidental ingestion of essential oils and the placement of products containing essential oil into the child's nasal cavity.

For this age group, it is still considered best practice to introduce children to one essential oil at a time. Using this simple method of introduction, you will be better able to monitor for adverse reactions and sensitivities and can more easily ascertain the culprit should such reactions occur. Once you are certain about the tolerability of the essential oils you would like to use with your child, it is recommended that when creating mixtures or blends, refrain from using more than three, but focus on using only two essential oils at a time.

Avoiding Eucalyptus and Peppermint with Children under Six

Although eucalyptus and peppermint essential oils can be incredibly supportive to the respiratory system, most aromatherapy and essential oil safety experts adamantly oppose their use on or around children under the age of six due to the presence of compounds that have led to nonfatal but severely toxic reactions in young children. These two compounds are menthol, in peppermint, and 1,8-cineole, in eucalyptus species (of which there are many). Essential oils high in menthol or 1,8-cineole can cause central nervous system and respiratory problems, notably a slowing of respiration rate. Although these problems have resulted only from accidental instillation into the nose, accidental ingestion, and the use of isolated compounds (isolated menthol, not peppermint essential oil, which contains some menthol), many aromatherapists take the stance that we are better safe than sorry. Essential oil safety experts have stated that not all essential oils containing 1,8-cineole or menthol are unsafe for children, but safe doses for menthol- and 1,8-cineole-containing essential oils for children under six have yet to be established. The following chart provides a list of essential oils high in menthol and 1,8-cineole that should likely be avoided for use with children under six and should never be applied to or near their faces. Keep in mind that there are a variety of eucalyptus species with various levels of 1,8-cineole. This list is not exhaustive but rather contains common essential oils that you may come across.

COMMON ESSENTIAL OILS
HIGH IN 1,8-CINEOLE AND MENTHOL

1,8-CINEOLE	Cardamom • Eucalyptus (all species) • Fragonia • Galangal • Ho leaf • Holy basil • Hyssop • Myrtle • Niaouli • Rosalina • Rosemary • White sage
MENTHOL	Cornmint • Lemon basil

OTHER ESSENTIAL OILS TO AVOID WITH CHILDREN UNDER SIX

+ Aniseed
+ Chaste tree (vitex)
+ Fennel, bitter or sweet
+ Star anise
+ Sweet birch
+ Wintergreen

Essential Oil Safety and Application Guidelines for Children Ages 6 to 12

As children grow older, their skin and internal systems become more robust, and essential oil choices and appropriate dilution ratios become less restrictive. The recommended dilution ratios for children ages 6 to 12 fall between 1.5 percent and 2 percent, which equates to 12 to 16 drops of essential oil per ounce of carrier or base. In some cases, for example, with older children in this age group who need stronger support, a 3 percent absolute maximum dilution (24 drops per ounce) is considered safe as long as it is applied for short periods of time (for example, one-off applications) and the essential oil is deemed safe for this age group. However, when using essential oils topically, dilutions toward the 1.5 percent end of the spectrum are more appropriate for younger children due to their smaller body size, with dilutions of 2 to 3 percent being more appropriate for older, larger children.

Your child's immune system has likely matured by this age, making adverse reactions from proper dilutions of essential oils not as likely. Using undiluted essential oils on the skin is not recommended, in order to avoid adverse skin reactions and sensitization. When introducing new essential oils topically, it is always a good idea to do a patch test first to establish any possible allergy or sensitivity. It is also important to remember to avoid the use of photosensitizing essential oils in topical applications if your child's skin is going to be exposed to sunlight after or between applications. When making blends, most aromatherapists keep it simple and use a maximum of three essential oils in any one blend.

By the time your child is six, peppermint and eucalyptus essential oils are not nearly as problematic to use. Although some essential oil safety experts recommend avoiding topical use of eucalyptus until a child is 10 years old, other aromatherapists deem topical use safe for children six and older if the appropriate dilutions and safety protocols are adhered to. For example, if you choose to use these essential oils on or around a child younger than 10, do not insert or allow the instillation of blends containing eucalyptus or peppermint essential oils into the child's nose, and refrain from using these oils on or near the face. Be mindful of not overdoing it, making sure to take breaks from these powerful oils, and using them only when their support is truly needed.

Aromatic use of essential oils remains the safest route. By the time a child is six years old, the amount of essential oils that can be used in a diffuser is generally the same as per the manufacturer's instructions. Diffusing fewer drops of essential oils for shorter periods of time and fewer times throughout the day is important if any of your children are still under the age of six. Otherwise, following the manufacturer's instructions and diffusing for 30 minutes at a time several times a day is likely safe. Although daily diffusion is considered unproblematic, taking breaks is always a good idea for the people in your home, for your pocketbook, and for the planet.

Direct inhalation using cotton balls or personal inhalers is also likely safe for this age group as long as your younger children are aware of how to use them and that they should never place them in the nose, ears, or mouth. With children younger than 10, it might be safest to supervise direct inhalation.

Essential Oil Safety and Application Guidelines for Children 12 and Older

Now that your child is 12 or older, safe essential oil choices and dilution ratios are similar to those for adults. Like with 6- to 12-year-olds, dilution ratios exist on a spectrum for this age group, ranging from 2 percent to 3 percent (16 to 24 drops per ounce) all the way to a maximum of 5 percent (36 drops per ounce) when stronger, short-term support is needed. However, the body of a 12-year-old may be smaller and less robust than that of an 18-year-old, so 2 percent dilutions are more appropriate for the younger age range. In fact, essential oil safety experts iterate that when considering dilution ratios for children 15 years and younger, the concentration of essential oils in topical full-body applications (for example, massage oils, body moisturizers, and baths) should be reduced according to the child's age and body size. Also, if your older teen is sensitive or suffers from allergies, skin conditions, or other medical problems, it is recommended that you use lower dilutions. Just because a child is older and bigger than they used to be, it doesn't mean they need higher doses of essential oils.

Special attention should be paid to dilution ratios and daily skin care. Although 2 percent to 3 percent is considered standard for this age group, this dilution generally refers to non-daily topical use. When working with daily skin care blends, it is important to stick with a maximum dilution of 1 percent (8 drops in 1 ounce) to avoid adverse skin reactions or the buildup of sensitivities, especially when working with blends intended for the face or other more sensitive areas. If your teen is using essential oils for facial skin care or cosmetics, it will be important to remind them not to overdo it. Too much essential oil use, especially on the face, can be counterproductive and irritating. Similarly, if a child is outside and exposed to sunlight, it will be important to avoid photosensitizing oils, which could cause significant sunburn. It is also recommended to change up your essential oil routine from time to time. Prepare a few different essential oil blends that provide similar support, and alternate their use every few weeks.

Certain essential oils deemed safe for this age group are "hotter" and more likely to burn the skin than others. These essential oils include ginger, oregano, black pepper, clove, thyme, and cinnamon bark or leaf, to name a few. It is best practice to use less of these and other strong essential oils for this age group. It is also best practice to use a weaker dilution ratio, for example not exceeding 0.5 percent total dilution for ginger, clove, or cinnamon bark, or making sure to use a maximum of 4 or 5 drops per ounce of carrier or base allocated for a 2 percent to 3 percent blend.

A 5 percent dilution ratio is the maximum safe concentration for topical aromatherapy applications that are being used on a one-off or short-term basis on small areas of skin. These applications may include home first aid blends for insect bites and stings, cosmetic blends for zits or ingrown hairs, or even personal perfumes. Regardless of the dilution ratio you are using, most aromatherapists use no more than three, or occasionally four, essential oils in any one blend.

Direct inhalation of essential oils can be incredibly useful and supportive for this age group. For example, a personal inhaler can be carried around in a purse or book bag for convenient, on-demand aromatherapy support. Aromatherapy jewelry can also be a wonderful tool. By this time in their lives, it is easier for your kids to understand and learn essential oil safety protocols and to employ these safe practices in their personal time. When diffusing essential oils in the home, follow the manufacturer's instructions for the appropriate amount of essential oil for your diffuser and diffuse only in 30- to 60-minute durations a few times a day. The dilution ratios for aromatherapy mists and sprays can follow those of topical application. Just make sure you are blending, misting, and diffusing responsibly, taking note of safe essential oils and dilution ratios that are inclusive of every member of your family.

Blends for Two to Six Years

SAFE ESSENTIAL OILS TO ADD TO YOUR LIST FOR CHILDREN
AGES 2 TO 6

+ Benzoin
+ Clary sage
+ Copaiba

+ Lemongrass
+ Lime
+ Melissa

+ Myrrh
+ Spearmint
+ Sweet basil

+ Vetiver
+ Yarrow
+ Ylang-ylang

Respiratory and Immune Support Diffusion Blend

CHILDREN 2+, TEENS, ADULTS, SENIORS

TO MAKE THE BLEND
Add the essential oils to a dark glass bottle with a dropper. Swirl the oils to blend. Cap the bottle tightly and be sure to label the blend. Store it in a cool, dark place away from the reach of young ones. Use it within 6 months of blending.

TO USE THE BLEND
Add the appropriate number of essential oil drops to a diffuser and diffuse for 30 minutes at a time several times a day. This blend can be used for several days in a row before a break from it is needed.

TIP: You can also add drops at the dilution appropriate for the age group to 1 to 2 ounces of distilled water and use as a room mist or linen spray. If spraying pillows, please note that the spray might stain lighter-color cases. Also make sure that it has had time to evaporate properly before coming in contact with your child's skin.

AROMATIC

MAKES ½ OUNCE

1 teaspoon thyme
    essential oil
1 teaspoon white pine
    essential oil
1 teaspoon benzoin
    essential oil

Stings and Bites Be Gone Salve

1% DILUTION

TO MAKE THE SALVE

Make sure to have a jar or salve tins ready. Gently heat the olive oil and beeswax in a double boiler or bain-marie until the beeswax is melted. Stir occasionally to ensure they are well mixed. Remove from heat and allow to cool until just warmer than body temperature (or the mixture is just beginning to solidify). Add the essential oils and stir until they are thoroughly blended. Pour or spoon the mixture into the prepared container(s). Label and store the salve in a cool, dark location. Use it within 12 months of blending.

TO USE THE SALVE

Using clean fingers or a cotton swab, apply a pea-sized or smaller amount of salve to a bite or sting. Cover with a bandage to avoid spreading around or being wiped off. Let sit for several hours before removing the bandage. If needed, clean the area with soap and water.

TOPICAL

MAKES 1½ CUPS

1¼ cups cold-pressed
   olive oil
¼ cup beeswax beads
   or shavings
25 drops myrrh essential oil
25 drops lavender
   essential oil
15 drops spearmint
   essential oil

TIP: Use a bit more beeswax for a harder salve and less beeswax for a softer salve. Avoid adding essential oils to a really hot oil-wax blend as they can evaporate and oxidize, which compromises the quality of your salve.

Take a Deep Breath Warming Chest Rub

CHILDREN 2+, TEENS, ADULTS, SENIORS

1% DILUTION

TOPICAL

MAKES ABOUT 1 CUP

TO MAKE THE RUB

Gently warm the coconut oil in a double boiler or bain-marie until it is soft enough to stir. Remove the coconut oil from heat and allow it to cool until it's just warmer than body temperature (or it's just beginning to solidify). It should be close to room temperature when adding essential oils. Add the essential oils and stir well. Transfer the rub to a glass jar with a tight-fitting lid, label it, store it in a cool, dark place, and use it within 6 to 12 months of blending.

TO USE THE RUB

Gently dip your clean index finger into the jar and scoop out a pea-sized dollop of the rub. Place the dollop in the palm of your hand and rub your hands together until they are warm and the rub is melted and evenly dispersed over your palms. With gentle, upward stroking motions, apply the rub to your child's chest, upper arms, and upper back. Do not apply the rub on or near your child's face or to areas that could come in contact with the eyes or mouth. Apply it two or three times a day as needed to support breathing.

1 cup unrefined coconut oil (solid at room temperature)
30 drops copaiba essential oil
30 drops frankincense essential oil
5 drops ginger essential oil

Bubble Gum Bubble Bath

CHILDREN 2+, TEENS, ADULTS, SENIORS

1% DILUTION

TO MAKE THE BUBBLE BATH

Add the liquid soap to a glass measuring cup. In a separate glass bowl, mix the olive oil and essential oils and stir well. Pour the mixture into the liquid soap and stir well. Pour the bubble bath into a 4-ounce PET-free plastic bottle with a pump and close the top tightly. Label and store the bubble bath in a cool, dark, place. Use it within 6 months of blending. Keep out of the reach of children.

TO USE THE BUBBLE BATH

Add a few squirts to warm, running bathwater and enjoy! Make sure the soap does not end up in your child's mouth or eyes.

TIP: You can store the bubble bath in a glass bottle, but the risk of shattering is high. You can also use some of this soap on a washcloth or sponge, making sure to avoid your child's face.

TOPICAL

MAKES ABOUT ½ CUP

6 tablespoons liquid castile soap or similar bubble bath base

2 tablespoons cold-pressed olive oil

12 drops grapefruit essential oil

10 drops mandarin essential oil

10 drops Roman chamomile essential oil

Bug Off Bug Spray

CHILDREN 2+, TEENS, ADULTS, SENIORS

1% DILUTION

TO MAKE THE SPRAY

Add the essential oils to a 1-ounce dark glass bottle with an aromatizer. Add the fractionated coconut oil, cap the bottle tightly, and shake vigorously. Make sure to label the spray. Store it in a cool, dark place, and use it within 6 months of blending.

TO USE THE SPRAY

Apply to the arms, chest, legs, and scalp, avoiding direct contact with the face and eyes. You can spray it into your hand and then rub it onto your child's skin and scalp. This spray can be reapplied several times over the course of the day.

TIP: This recipe can be made at stronger essential oil concentrations for older children and adults. Be prepared that it is greasy until absorbed into the skin and may temporarily stain clothes. Be mindful that lemongrass essential oil is photosensitizing, so any skin that has been sprayed should be kept out of direct sunlight. If you are concerned about photosensitization, try using rose geranium essential oil instead.

TOPICAL, PHOTOSENSITIZING

MAKES 1 OUNCE

4 drops lemongrass essential oil

4 drops patchouli essential oil

2 tablespoons fractionated coconut oil

Bumps and Bruises Balm

CHILDREN 2+, TEENS, ADULTS, SENIORS

1% DILUTION

TO MAKE THE BALM

Add the aloe vera gel to a glass jar with a tight-fitting lid. Add the essential oils and vitamin E oil and stir well. Cap the jar tightly, label, and store the balm in the refrigerator. Use it within 3 to 6 months of blending. If signs of mold or odd smells appear, discard and make a fresh batch.

TO USE THE BALM

Do not apply to broken skin. Using a clean finger or cotton swab, dab a small amount of balm to the area of need and rub it gently into the skin. Apply several times a day. Do not use on or near your child's face.

TOPICAL

MAKES ABOUT ½ CUP

½ cup aloe vera gel
10 drops lavender
   essential oil
10 drops yarrow essential oil
12 drops Roman or German
   chamomile essential oil
10 drops vitamin E oil

Blends for 6 to 12 Years

SAFE ESSENTIAL OILS TO ADD TO YOUR LIST FOR CHILDREN
AGES 6 TO 12

- Bay laurel
- Blue gum eucalyptus
- Coriander
- Helichrysum
- Lemon eucalyptus
- Myrtle
- Niaouli
- Peppermint
- Rosemary
- Sweet fennel

Super Snotty Diffuser or Facial Steam Blend

CHILDREN 6+, TEENS, ADULTS, SENIORS

TO MAKE THE BLEND

Add the essential oils to a dark glass bottle with a dropper. Swirl the oils to blend. Cap the bottle tightly and be sure to label it clearly. Store the blend in a cool, dark place, and use it within 6 months of blending. Keep away from the reach of young ones.

TO USE THE BLEND

Add the appropriate number of essential oil drops to a diffuser (not more than 3 to 5 drops per 100 milliliters of water) and diffuse for 30 minutes at a time several times a day. Alternatively, you can use this blend as a steam. Heat water on the stove until steaming but not boiling. Carefully pour the water into a large glass bowl and add 1 or 2 drops of the blend. Sit close by as your child, *with eyes closed*, holds their head over the steam for 30 seconds at a time, stopping to breathe fresh air and blow or wipe their nose. Cover your child's head and the bowl with a towel for a more concentrated effect. This blend can be used twice a day for several days in a row before a break from it is needed.

AROMATIC

MAKES ½ OUNCE

1½ teaspoons myrtle essential oil

1 teaspoon white pine essential oil

½ teaspoon peppermint essential oil

TIP: Make sure your child's eyes are closed during a facial steam. Alternatively, add drops at the dilution appropriate for the age group to 1 to 2 ounces of distilled water and use as a room mist or linen spray. Make sure that it has had time to evaporate properly before coming in contact with your child's skin.

Settle Down Room Mist

CHILDREN 6+, TEENS, ADULTS, SENIORS

2% DILUTION

TO MAKE THE SPRAY

Add the essential oils to a 2-ounce glass bottle with an aromatizer and swirl the oils to blend. Fill the bottle with the distilled water, cap it tightly, and shake it vigorously. Don't forget to label the bottle. Store the spray in a cool, dark place away from the reach of children. Use it within 6 months of blending.

TO USE THE SPRAY

Shake vigorously before use. Spray 2 or 3 pumps around an unsettled room. You can also use it on a pillow before bed. For dispersed coverage, make sure your pillow is at least 1 foot away. This spray may stain white pillowcases. Avoid spraying in faces and eyes.

AROMATIC

MAKES 2 OUNCES

5 drops clary sage
  essential oil
5 drops ylang-ylang
  essential oil
3 drops vetiver essential oil
3 drops sweet orange
  essential oil (or another
  citrus essential oil, such
  as grapefruit, mandarin,
  lemon, or lime)
2 tablespoons distilled water

Soothe My Angry Skin Lotion

CHILDREN 6+, TEENS, ADULTS, SENIORS

1% DILUTION

TO MAKE THE LOTION

In a glass measuring cup, combine the base cream, vitamin E oil, and essential oils and stir well. Spoon the lotion into a glass jar with a tight-fitting lid. Label and store the jar in a cool, dark location or in the refrigerator. Use the lotion within 6 months of blending.

TO USE THE LOTION

Apply the lotion to inflamed, irritated areas of skin as needed to support relief. This lotion is safe for daily use. Please remember that using essential oil blends on irritated or inflamed skin increases the risk for adverse skin reactions. Do not apply to your child's face.

TOPICAL

MAKES ABOUT 1 CUP

1 cup base cream or
  aloe vera gel
10 drops vitamin E oil
25 drops helichrysum
  essential oil
25 drops lavender
  essential oil
15 drops German chamomile
  essential oil

Focus Blend Roll-On

2% DILUTION

TO MAKE THE BLEND

Add the essential oils to a roller bottle and gently swirl the oils together. Fill the bottle with the olive oil, and close it with the rollerball and cap. Shake it well. Store the blend in a cool, dark place, and use it within 6 months of blending.

TO USE THE BLEND

Allow your child to gently dab the roller on their inner wrists and sniff them when needed to maintain focus. When children are mature enough to use an aromatherapy roller on their own, teach them how to use the aromatherapy roller safely at school as needed, if allowed. Use several times a day to support settled learning.

TIP: If your child refuses to participate while at home, use the roller on your own wrists when you sit with them for homework or homeschooling time.

AROMATIC, TOPICAL

MAKES ABOUT ½ OUNCE

- 4 drops bay laurel essential oil
- 2 drops rosemary essential oil
- 2 drops lemon essential oil
- 1 tablespoon cold-pressed olive oil or fractionated coconut oil

Wound Aftercare Healing Support Gel

CHILDREN 6+, TEENS, ADULTS, SENIORS

1% DILUTION

TO MAKE THE LOTION

Add the aloe vera gel and essential oils to a glass measuring cup and mix well. Spoon the lotion into a glass jar with a tight-fitting lid. Label and store the jar in the refrigerator for up to 3 months.

TO USE THE LOTION

Do not apply the lotion to broken skin, which could be susceptible to adverse reactions. At a dilution of 1 percent, this lotion is safe for daily use until no longer needed. Do not apply to your child's face.

TOPICAL

MAKES ABOUT 1 CUP

- 1 cup aloe vera gel
- 25 drops helichrysum essential oil
- 25 drops lavender essential oil
- 15 drops niaouli essential oil

Spring Pollen Immune Support Diffuser Blend

TO MAKE THE BLEND

Add the essential oils to a dark glass bottle with a dropper. Swirl the oils to blend. Label and store the bottle in a cool, dark place, and use it within 6 months of blending. Keep it away from the reach of young ones.

TO USE THE BLEND

Add the appropriate number of essential oil drops to a diffuser and diffuse for 30 minutes at a time several times a day for a maximum of one week before taking a break. If essential oils are irritating to any family members' respiratory allergies, stop using them.

AROMATIC

MAKES ½ OUNCE

1½ teaspoons frankincense essential oil

1 teaspoon white pine essential oil

½ teaspoon blue gum eucalyptus essential oil

Blends for 12+ Years

SAFE ESSENTIAL OILS TO ADD TO YOUR LIST FOR CHILDREN
AGES 12+

- ✦ Caraway
- ✦ Cardamom
- ✦ Carrot seed
- ✦ Cypress
- ✦ Nutmeg
- ✦ Palmarosa
- ✦ Sage
- ✦ Valerian

I Love My Face Oil Cleanser

CHILDREN 12+, TEENS, ADULTS, SENIORS
1% DILUTION

TO MAKE THE OIL CLEANSER

Add the essential oils to a dark glass bottle with a pump.
Swirl the oils to mix. Add the jojoba and hazelnut oils, cap
the bottle, and shake it vigorously. Label and store the
blend in a cool, dark place, and use it within 6 months of
blending.

TO USE THE OIL CLEANSER

Apply 1 small pump of oil cleanser to dry skin using
your fingertips and gently massage the face and neck
for several minutes. Dampen a facial towel with warm
water, and wipe away excess oil cleanser. Follow up with
Fab Facial Toner (see page 70). This blend is safe for
daily use.

TIP: When skin is oily and/or troublesome, some teens may
find the idea of using an oil cleanser unappealing. Although
oil cleansing works well for some, it may not work well for
others. Your teen will know after a month or so if it is a helpful, supportive practice for their skin. This oil cleanser can be
used as a moisturizer in lieu of being used for cleansing.

TOPICAL

MAKES 2 OUNCES

4 drops cypress essential oil
2 drops German chamomile
essential oil
2 drops palmarosa
essential oil
2 tablespoons jojoba oil
2 tablespoons hazelnut oil

Bye-Bye Body Odor Spray

CHILDREN 12+, TEENS, ADULTS, SENIORS

1% DILUTION

TO MAKE THE SPRAY

Add the essential oils to a dark glass bottle with an aromatizer. Add the magnesium oil, witch hazel, and lavender hydrosol and shake the bottle vigorously until blended. Label and store the spray in a cool, dark place for up to 3 months.

TO USE THE SPRAY

Apply a couple spritzes under each arm after bathing. This blend is safe for daily use.

TIP: You can adjust the amount of magnesium oil used in this blend to suit the needs of the individual. On its own, magnesium oil can sting or slightly irritate the skin but is very effective at neutralizing body odor. If this blend needs more odor-eliminating power, try increasing the amount of magnesium oil to 2 tablespoons and reducing the witch hazel and lavender hydrosol. For a more masculine scent, try replacing the rose geranium essential oil with spruce or fir and replacing the lavender essential oil with sweet marjoram or bay laurel.

TOPICAL

MAKES 2 OUNCES

5 drops rose geranium
   essential oil
5 drops cypress essential oil
6 drops lavender essential oil
1 tablespoon magnesium oil
1 tablespoon witch hazel
2 tablespoons lavender
   hydrosol or distilled water

Sore Winner Sports Rub for Muscles and Joints

CHILDREN 12+, TEENS, ADULTS

4% DILUTION

TO MAKE THE RUB

Gently warm the coconut oil in a double boiler or bain-marie until it is soft enough to stir. Remove the coconut oil from heat and allow it to cool until it's just warmer than body temperature (or just beginning to solidify). Thoroughly blend in the essential oils. Scoop the rub into a glass jar with a tight-fitting lid and label it. Store the jar in a cool, dark place. Use the rub within 6 to 12 months of blending if using coconut oil, or 3 to 6 months if using aloe vera gel (aloe vera gel should not be heated).

TO USE THE RUB

Apply to muscles or joints as needed. Make sure to wash hands after use. At a 4 percent dilution, it is best practice to use as temporary support only. Avoid daily use.

TIP: For a less greasy rub, use aloe vera gel instead of coconut oil.

TOPICAL

MAKES ¼ CUP

¼ cup unrefined coconut oil (solid at room temperature) or aloe vera gel

30 drops rosemary essential oil

20 drops black pepper essential oil

14 drops ginger essential oil or clove essential oil

Fab Facial Toner

CHILDREN 12+, TEENS, ADULTS, SENIORS

TO MAKE THE FACIAL TONER

Add all the ingredients to a 2-ounce dark glass bottle with an aromatizer, close it tightly, and shake well. Label and store the bottle in a cool, dark place or in the refrigerator, and use it within 3 months.

TO USE THE FACIAL TONER

After cleansing, apply the toner on the face and neck with a spritzer or a cotton facial pad. Pat skin dry and apply a moisturizer. This toner is safe for daily use.

TOPICAL

MAKES 2 OUNCES

1 tablespoon witch hazel distillate

1 tablespoon rose hydrosol

1 tablespoon German chamomile hydrosol

1 tablespoon yarrow hydrosol

Calm and Collected Personal Inhaler Blend

TO MAKE THE BLEND

Add the essential oils to a small, dark glass bottle. Swirl the oils to blend. Cap the bottle tightly and be sure to label the blend. Store it in a cool, dark place, and use it within 6 months of blending.

TO USE THE BLEND

Add 10 to 15 drops to the wick of an aromatherapy inhaler and use it as needed. Similarly, you can add 1 or 2 drops to aromatherapy jewelry, a cotton ball, or a facial tissue to carry with you to use as needed. Or you can add 15 to 30 drops to 1 ounce of distilled water to use as an aromatherapy mist. If using an aromatherapy diffuser, follow the manufacturer's instructions regarding the number of essential oil drops to use per diffusion. Diffuse for 30 to 60 minutes at a time one or two times a day.

TIP: Although very calming, the aroma of valerian is not for everybody. Both patchouli and vetiver essential oils are also considered grounding and calming and can be used in place of valerian. Involve your teen in essential oil choices, sitting together and working on a blend that is pleasing to them.

AROMATIC

MAKES ½ OUNCE

1½ teaspoons clary sage essential oil

1 teaspoon sweet basil essential oil

½ teaspoon valerian essential oil or nutmeg essential oil

Cram for Exams Study Blend for Diffusion or Personal Inhalers

CHILDREN 12+, TEENS, ADULTS, SENIORS

TO MAKE THE BLEND

Add the essential oils to a small, dark glass bottle. Swirl the oils to blend. Cap the bottle tightly and be sure to label the blend. Store it in a cool, dark place, and use it within 6 months of blending.

TO USE THE BLEND

Add 10 to 15 drops to the wick of an aromatherapy inhaler and use as needed. Similarly, you can add 1 or 2 drops to aromatherapy jewelry, a cotton ball, or a facial tissue to carry with you to use as needed. Or you can add 15 to 30 drops to 1 ounce of distilled water to use as an aromatherapy mist. If using an aromatherapy diffuser, follow the manufacturer's instructions regarding the number of essential oil drops to use per diffusion. Diffuse for 30 to 60 minutes at a time one or two times a day.

AROMATIC

MAKES ½ OUNCE

1½ teaspoons rosemary essential oil

1 teaspoon sweet basil essential oil

½ teaspoon sage essential oil

Scar Tissue Healing Support Blend

CHILDREN 12+, TEENS, ADULTS, SENIORS

4% DILUTION

TO MAKE THE BLEND

Add the essential oils to a dark glass bottle with a dropper. Swirl the oils to blend. Add the vitamin E oil, rosehip seed oil, and St. John's wort herbal-infused oil. Cap the bottle tightly and shake it vigorously until blended. Label and store the blend in a cool, dark place. Use it within 6 months of blending.

TO USE THE BLEND

Apply to small areas of the skin that need extra healing support. Although this blend is 4 percent dilution, if used on small areas it can be used daily. Avoid using this blend on large areas of the body on a daily basis. This blend can be used on small areas of skin on the face and neck, but be mindful to avoid direct contact with eyes, ears, and other sensitive membranes.

TIP: If you can't find herbal-infused oils, you can learn to make your own. Alternatively, substitute argan oil for either herbal-infused oil.

TOPICAL

MAKES ABOUT 1 OUNCE

16 drops carrot seed essential oil

10 drops frankincense essential oil

10 drops helichrysum essential oil

10 drops vitamin E oil

1 tablespoon rosehip seed oil

1 tablespoon St. John's wort herbal-infused oil or gotu kola herbal-infused oil

SAFETY TIPS

✦ Pay careful attention to each age group's safe dilution ratios. For children 15 years and younger, concentrations of essential oils should be reduced according to their body size.

✦ Remember that irritated, inflamed, or broken skin is more susceptible to adverse skin reactions and sensitization to essential oils.

✦ If essential oil comes in contact with the eyes, flush with any type of high-quality vegetable oil. Vegetable oil will dissolve the essential oil, whereas water will only disperse it and might make it worse.

✦ If using photosensitizing essential oils in bug sprays, moisturizing lotions, or other topical applications, remember to avoid direct contact with sunlight.

✦ Certain essential oils, such as oregano, cinnamon, and clove, are "hotter" than others. You will need to use less of these potent essential oils in your blends.

✦ Especially with children under the age of 10, make sure to patch-test essential oils before using them on large areas of the skin.

✦ Peppermint and eucalyptus essential oils should be avoided topically and aromatically with children under six.

✦ When diffusing or misting essential oils, make sure you are using essential oils and blending to dilutions that are appropriate to all age groups in your family.

TIPS FOR TEENS

✦ Less is more. Be mindful to not overdo it with essential oils. Do not use essential oils in a way that will negatively impact others.

✦ Give your skin time to get used to essential oils, but stop using them if further irritation occurs.

✦ Blend oils for yourself that are appealing to you.

✦ Do not expose your skin to sunlight if you have been using photosensitizing essential oils.

BEST PRACTICES

✦ Take breaks from home diffusion and misting. Although daily aromatic use of essential oils is considered safe, it is best practice to take breaks from time to time, especially if you are also using essential oils in personal care and cleaning products
or are exposed to them in different ways throughout the day.

✦ Avoid using more than two or three essential oils in any one blend, and change up your blends from time to time to avoid building up sensitivities.

MY NOTES

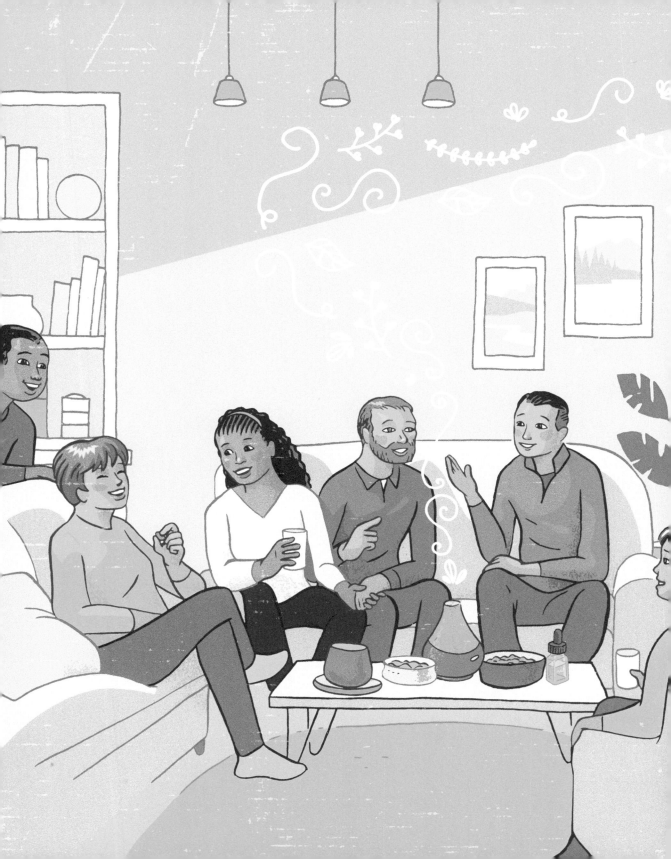

Chapter Five

ESSENTIAL OILS
FOR ADULTS

Journey into Adulthood

Being an adult in our modern Western society is full of physical, emotional, and spiritual challenges. From the age of 18 onward, it is as if we leap from one set of pressures, failures, and accomplishments to the next: graduating from school, finding (and sometimes losing) our dream job, getting married, and starting a family of our own. Before we know it, credit card bills and mortgages have piled up on top of car and college loan payments. As we age, our families grow and, with them, the demands of hungry bellies and hopes of providing all the resources our children need to get ahead and fulfill their dreams. By the time we reach our mid-50s, we have had decades full of joy, sadness, excitement, boredom, frustration, and relief—all of this is just in time for major transitions in our bodies and our sense of self as the evolution from adulthood into elderhood begins.

Benefits of Essential Oils for Adults

Stress seems to come from all directions, adding to the difficulties of managing our health and nurturing our well-being. Indeed, stress is now considered a major force behind many chronic health problems. High blood pressure, heart disease, and difficulties maintaining healthy cholesterol and blood sugar levels are now understood to be rooted in chronic stress. Health problems in and of themselves are stressful, and it is all too easy to succumb to the cyclical nature of ill health and the harmful impact of unrelenting stressors.

Women and men embody both adulthood and stress differently; male and female bodies are presented with different sets of challenges based on our divergent biology and socially constructed gender roles. Even the sources and impacts of stress can present unique challenges to our health and well-being. For example, in one cross-sectional study of almost 3,000 people between the ages of 18 and 65, women listed health and family-related events as sources of stress more frequently than men, whereas men listed relationships, finances, and work-related events as their key stressors. In this same study, women scored significantly higher than men on physical and psychological symptoms of stress, such as anxiety and depression, headaches, insomnia, and chronic pain, leading researchers to the conclusion that women and men suffer through stress and express its impacts differently.

Stress is also related to the impacts of poor nutrition, not drinking enough water, and a sedentary lifestyle. In fact, stress researchers emphasize that an adequate balance between energy expenditure and growth and healing processes is fundamental to long-term health. From this perspective, the diseases of modern society are more likely a result of the lack of rest, recovery, and restitution than they are of the levels of stress itself.

Supporting the stressed-out body, mind, and spirit in achieving rest and recuperation is where aromatherapy really shines. Whether it helps with processing emotions, supporting pain relief, or encouraging you to breathe more deeply, essential oils can play a critical role in restoring balance between the demands of adulthood and the needs of being human.

When trapped in cycles of imbalance, taking care of our bodies, our emotional selves, and even our spirits can seem impossible—especially when we are raising families and the needs and well-being of others always seem to come before our own. Procuring and cooking nutritious food can become too expensive or effortful; exercise, too time-consuming or exhausting. Although aromatherapy and essential oils can support you physically, emotionally, and spiritually, they cannot make everything alright on their own. In fact, incorporating aromatherapy safely into your life requires that you acknowledge its limitations and prioritize proper nutrition, hydration, movement, and relaxation as much as you possibly can.

Essential Oil Safety Considerations for Ages 18 to 55

Throughout the preceding chapters in this book, we have thoroughly reviewed safety considerations and best practices for the topical and aromatic use of essential oils for various age groups and life stages. Please refer back to chapter 1 (see page 6) for an overview of all relevant safety precautions. Safety protocols and application guidelines remain the same for individuals in your family who are ages 18 to 55: continue to use patch tests when introducing new essential oils, do not blend with toxic or potentially hazardous oils, avoid undiluted use of essential oils directly on the skin or sensitive membranes, remain cognizant of potential skin irritants and photosensitizers, and take breaks from time to time. However, there is one safety consideration that has yet to be explored, which concerns the potential for essential oils to interfere with your prescription medications.

Some essential oils and essential oil components have been studied in regard to their potential to interact with specific pharmaceutical drugs. Most of these studies have been conducted using research models and methods that do not accurately depict levels of exposure or modes of application that one would find with topical and aromatic use of essential oils in humans. Much of the concern regarding the topical or aromatic use of essential oils and drug interactions is therefore theoretical, and essential oil safety experts recognize very little risk of interactions when essential oils are used in this way.

However, there have been several case reports regarding extensive topical use of preparations containing high levels of the essential oil component methyl salicylate enhancing the effects of the anticoagulants warfarin and heparin, which led to extensive bleeding and hemorrhaging. Methyl salicylate is found in significant quantities in wintergreen and sweet birch essential oils, both of which have been listed as "potentially hazardous" in this book and whose use has been advised against. Therefore, further caution is advised with the topical use of essential oils high in methyl salicylate, such as wintergreen or sweet birch, especially if you are currently taking anticoagulants.

In addition, many common components of essential oils have demonstrated the capacity to enhance drug absorption via the skin, which could lead to toxic outcomes. If you are on prescribed medications that are delivered via skin patches, essential oil safety experts recommend to not use essential oils on the skin near, adjacent to, or under conventional drug patches.

Although essential oils used topically or aromatically are unlikely to interfere with pharmaceuticals, internal and oral use of essential oils can pose a more significant interaction risk. Mechanisms behind these interactions could include enhancing or reducing the effect of the medication or inducing or inhibiting a drug's metabolism. These latter possibilities can result in either drug toxicity caused by heightened levels of a drug in the system or therapeutic failure of a drug as a result of insufficient levels of the drug in the system. The degree of risk for these types of interactions are dependent upon the essential oil in question, the amount and timing of its ingestion, and the nature of the pharmaceutical being taken concurrently. Internal and oral use of essential oils has not been explored or recommended in this book, and the heightened risk of drug interactions emphasizes the need to work with a qualified health professional if you are considering using essential oils in this way.

Dilution ratios for topical use of essential oils with adults ages 18 to 55 are similar for those of older children and teens, with standard dilutions ranging from 2 to 2.5 percent (16 to 20 drops per ounce of carrier or base) and maxing out at 5 percent (36 drops per ounce) for blends of short-term use on small areas of the skin.

SAFE ESSENTIAL OILS TO ADD TO YOUR LIST FOR ADULTS AGES 18+

+ Angelica root

+ Catnip

+ Cistus

+ Galbanum

+ Hops

+ Inula

+ Jasmine

+ Tuberose

Recipes for Common Conundrums

Supple Skin Face Mask

TEENS, ADULTS, SENIORS

1% DILUTION

TO MAKE THE FACE MASK

Using a spice grinder or coffee grinder, grind the green tea and rolled oats until they are a fine power. In a glass bowl, mix the bentonite clay with the green tea and oat powder until evenly mixed. In a separate glass bowl, combine the jojoba oil, vitamin E oil, and essential oils and stir until blended. Slowly add the oil mixture to the dry ingredients, stirring until the mixture has a smooth, even texture and there are no lumps. Scoop the mixture into a glass jar with a tight-fitting lid. Label and store the jar in the refrigerator. Use it within 3 months of blending.

TO USE THE FACE MASK

Steam your face for several minutes over warm water, placing a towel over your head to concentrate the heat and open the pores. Pat the skin dry. Place 1 teaspoon of face mask powder in a small dish. Slowly stir in drops of water until you achieve a smooth-paste consistency. Gently spread a thin layer of mask over the face and neck, avoiding delicate skin around the eyes and mouth. Keep the mask on until dry or almost dry. To remove, rinse with lukewarm water. Pat the skin dry and follow up with facial toner and moisturizer.

TOPICAL

MAKES ABOUT 1 CUP

1 teaspoon loose-leaf
  green tea
¼ cup organic rolled oats
½ cup bentonite or
  kaolin clay
1 teaspoon jojoba oil or
  cold-pressed olive oil
10 drops vitamin E oil
20 drops carrot seed
  essential oil
20 drops rose geranium
  essential oil
14 drops palmarosa
  essential oil
10 drops rosemary
  essential oil

Tired But Wired Soaking Salt

TEENS, ADULTS

2% DILUTION

TOPICAL

MAKES ABOUT ½ CUP

TO MAKE THE SOAKING SALT

In a glass measuring cup, combine all the essential oils and the sesame oil and mix well. Add the Epsom salt and thoroughly blend all ingredients together. Spoon the mixture into a glass jar, close with a tight-fitting lid, and label the soaking salt. Store the jar in a cool, dark place, and use it within 6 months of blending.

TO USE THE SOAKING SALT

Add ¼ cup of the soaking salt to warm, running bath-water. Soak for 10 to 15 minutes or until you feel relaxed and able to sleep.

TIP: Hops essential oil can be sensitizing to some individuals. It is recommended to perform a patch test before using this oil on large areas of the body. If sensitization occurs, nutmeg essential oil or ylang-ylang essential oil makes a nice substitute.

25 drops clary sage essential oil

25 drops vetiver essential oil

14 drops hops essential oil or ylang-ylang essential oil

1 tablespoon cold-pressed sesame oil or St. John's wort herbal-infused oil

½ cup Epsom salt

Stuck Circulation Support Gel

TEENS, ADULTS, SENIORS

2% DILUTION

TOPICAL

MAKES ABOUT ½ CUP

TO MAKE THE GEL

In a small bowl, combine the aloe vera gel and the essential oils and mix well. Transfer the gel to a small jar with a tight-fitting lid. Label and store the jar in a cool, dark place, and use it within 1 month of blending.

TO USE THE GEL

Gently dab small amounts on swollen or sore veins and hemorrhoids as needed up to three times a day.

½ cup aloe vera gel

20 drops rosemary essential oil

20 drops rose geranium essential oil

14 drops cedarwood essential oil

10 drops yarrow essential oil

Immune Support for Colds and Flus Personal Inhaler or Diffusion Blend

CHILDREN 12+, TEENS, ADULTS, SENIORS

TO MAKE THE BLEND

Add the essential oils to a small, dark glass dropper bottle. Swirl the oils to blend. Cap the bottle tightly and label the blend. Store it in a cool, dark place, and use it within 6 months of blending.

TO USE THE BLEND

Apply 10 to 15 drops to the wick of an aromatherapy inhaler; 1 to 2 drops to aromatherapy jewelry, a cotton ball, or a facial tissue; or 15 to 30 drops to 1 ounce of distilled water to use as an aromatherapy mist. If using an aromatherapy diffuser, follow the manufacturer's instructions regarding the number of essential oil drops to use per diffusion. Diffuse for 30 to 60 minutes one or two times a day.

AROMATIC

MAKES ½ OUNCE

1½ teaspoons cypress essential oil

1 teaspoon thyme essential oil

½ teaspoon inula essential oil

Irritable Belly Massage Blend

TEENS, ADULTS

TO MAKE THE BLEND

Add the essential oils to a dark glass bottle with a dropper. Swirl the oils to blend. Add the sesame oil, cap it tightly, and shake the bottle vigorously until blended. Label and store the blend in a cool, dark place. Use it within 6 months of blending.

TO USE THE BLEND

Place a few drops in your hand or directly on your lower abdomen and massage in a clockwise direction until absorbed. Can also be dabbed on the wrists or solar plexus or behind the ears to provide relaxing support to the digestive system.

2.5% DILUTION

TOPICAL

MAKES 1 OUNCE

10 drops peppermint essential oil

5 drops sweet fennel essential oil

5 drops catnip essential oil

2 tablespoons cold-pressed sesame oil

Open the Floodgates Facial Steam for Sinus Support

TO MAKE THE BLEND

Add all the essential oils to a dark glass bottle with a dropper. Swirl the oils to blend and cap it tightly. Label and store the bottle in a cool, dark place. Use it within 6 months of blending.

TO USE THE BLEND

Heat a pot of water on the stove until steaming but not boiling. Carefully pour the water into a large glass bowl. Add 3 to 5 drops of the blend into the hot water and sit with your head over the steam for 30 to 60 seconds at a time *with your eyes closed*, stopping to breathe fresh air and blow your nose. Cover your head and bowl with a towel for a more concentrated effect. This blend can be used twice a day for several days in a row before a break from it is needed. Alternatively, add the appropriate number of essential oil drops to a diffuser and diffuse for 30 to 60 minutes at a time several times a day.

AROMATIC

MAKES ½ OUNCE

1½ teaspoons lavender
   essential oil
1 teaspoon myrtle
   essential oil
½ teaspoon eucalyptus
   essential oil

TIP: To protect your eyes, make sure they are closed when doing a facial steam. If the number of drops in the steam seems too strong or feels irritating, reduce the number of drops and try again. You can also add drops at a 5 percent dilution to 1 to 2 ounces of distilled water (36 drops in 1 ounce or 72 drops in 2 ounces) and use as a room mist.

Crampy Crabby Periods Abdominal Hot Pack

TEENS, ADULTS

2.5% DILUTION

TO MAKE THE BLEND

Add the essential oils to a dark glass bottle with a dropper. Swirl the oils to blend. Add the castor oil, cap it tightly, and shake the bottle vigorously until mixed. Label and store the blend in a cool, dark place, and use it within 6 months of blending.

TO USE THE BLEND

Place a few drops in your hand or directly on your lower abdomen and massage in a clockwise direction until absorbed. Place a towel over your lower abdomen, followed by an electric heating pad or hot water bottle. Allow the heat to penetrate for 10 to 15 minutes. If well tolerated, repeat up to three times daily as needed.

TIP: Not everyone is comfortable using castor oil. Feel free to substitute olive oil or other preferred nut or seed oil. Remember that skin permeability increases with heat, and your skin may be more sensitive to essential oils when being coadministered with heating pads or hot water bottles. If the area of application begins to feel irritated, remove heat and promptly wash the abdomen with soap and water.

TOPICAL

MAKES 1 OUNCE

10 drops patchouli
   essential oil
5 drops ginger essential oil
5 drops hops essential oil
2 tablespoons castor oil

Loose and Nimble Joint and Muscle Rub

TO MAKE THE RUB

Gently warm the coconut oil in a double boiler or bain-marie until it is soft enough to stir (aloe vera gel should not be heated). Remove the coconut oil from heat and allow it to cool until it's just warmer than body temperature (or it's just beginning to solidify). It should be close to room temperature when adding essential oils. Add the cayenne pepper powder (if using) and the essential oils and stir well to blend. Scoop the rub into a glass jar with a tight-fitting lid, and label it. Store the jar in a cool, dark place, and use it within 6 to 12 months if using coconut oil or 3 to 6 months if using aloe vera gel.

TO USE THE RUB

Apply to muscles or joints as needed. Make sure to wash hands after use. This blend is safe for daily use.

TIP: Cayenne pepper can be found in the spice section at your local grocery store. This herb is traditionally used as a counterirritant to support a healthy inflammatory response. If you choose to use cayenne, expect an increased warming sensation and possible redness. If irritation or burning occurs, discontinue use. Wash your hands after application. Once you are comfortable using cayenne powder in this way, you can adjust the amount in the recipe as needed. However, refrain from using more than 1 teaspoon per cup for safety reasons.

TOPICAL

MAKES ABOUT 1 CUP

1 cup unrefined coconut oil (solid at room temperature) or aloe vera gel

¼ teaspoon cayenne pepper powder (optional)

40 drops ginger essential oil

40 drops clove essential oil

40 drops peppermint essential oil

Quitting Smoking/Sobriety Support Blend Personal Inhaler

TEENS, ADULTS, SENIORS

TO MAKE THE BLEND

Add the essential oils to a small, dark glass bottle. Swirl the oils to blend and cap it tightly. Label and store the blend in a cool, dark place, and use it within 6 months of blending.

TO USE THE BLEND

Apply 10 to 15 drops to the wick of an aromatherapy inhaler and use for support through cravings. Similarly, you can apply 1 or 2 drops to aromatherapy jewelry, a cotton ball, or a facial tissue to carry with you to use as needed. You can also add 15 to 30 drops to 1 ounce of distilled water to use as an aromatherapy mist, shaking well before use. If using an aromatherapy diffuser, follow the manufacturer's instructions regarding the number of essential oil drops to use per diffusion. Diffuse for 30 to 60 minutes at a time one or two times a day.

AROMATIC

MAKES ½ OUNCE

1½ teaspoons galbanum essential oil

1 teaspoon cistus essential oil

½ teaspoon sage essential oil

Building Intimacy Massage Blend

ADULTS, SENIORS

2% DILUTION

TO MAKE MASSAGE OIL

Add the essential oils to a dark glass bottle with a pump or dropper, and fill the bottle with the olive oil. Close it tightly and shake well. Label and store the massage oil in a cool, dark place, and use it within 3 months of blending.

TO USE MASSAGE OIL

This oil can be used for intimate massage. Do not use as a lubricant, as it could be irritating to sensitive membranes. Also avoid contact with latex condoms, as essential oils can impact their integrity.

TOPICAL

MAKES 2 OUNCES

15 drops vetiver essential oil

10 drops mandarin essential oil

7 drops jasmine essential oil

¼ cup cold-pressed olive oil or other nut or vegetable oil

Energetic and Motivated Roll-On Blend

TEENS, ADULTS, SENIORS

TO MAKE THE BLEND

Combine the essential oils in a roller bottle and gently swirl the oils together. Fill the bottle to the top with fractionated coconut oil. Close it with the rollerball and cap, and shake well. Label and store the bottle in a cool, dark place, and use it within 6 months of blending.

TO USE THE BLEND

Gently dab on the inner wrists, solar plexus, or heart chakra and/or behind your ears as needed when feeling like you need a pick-me-up.

TOPICAL

MAKES ½ OUNCE

10 drops sweet basil
    essential oil

4 drops bay laurel
    essential oil

4 drops grapefruit
    essential oil

1 tablespoon fractionated
    coconut oil or
    cold-pressed sesame oil

Release the Vice Roll-On for Temple Massage

CHILDREN 6+, TEENS, ADULTS, SENIORS

5% DILUTION

TO MAKE THE BLEND

Combine the essential oils in a roller bottle and gently swirl the oils together. Fill the bottle to the top with the fractionated coconut oil. Close it with the rollerball and cap, and shake well. Label and store the bottle in a cool, dark place, and use it within 6 months of blending.

TO USE THE BLEND

Gently dab on and massage the temples as needed to support relaxation. You can also use it on the inner wrists, solar plexus, or heart chakra and/or behind your ears as needed when feeling overwhelmed.

TOPICAL, AROMATIC

MAKES ½ OUNCE

10 drops rosemary
    essential oil

4 drops German chamomile
    essential oil

4 drops sweet orange
    essential oil

1 tablespoon fractionated
    coconut oil or
    cold-pressed sesame oil

Cooling the Flames Aromatherapy Mist

ADULTS, SENIORS

2.5% DILUTION

TO MAKE THE MIST

Combine all the essential oils in a dark glass bottle with an aromatizer. Fill the bottle the rest of the way with the distilled water, close it tightly, and shake vigorously. Label the bottle and carry it with you for on-demand cooling effects, but avoid leaving it in hot cars or direct sunlight. Use the mist within 3 months of blending.

TO USE THE MIST

Hold the bottle 1 foot away from your body and mist the back and front of your neck, chest, and face as needed for cooling support through hot flashes and night sweats.

TOPICAL, AROMATIC

MAKES 1 OUNCE

15 drops spearmint essential oil

10 drops sage essential oil

5 drops rose otto essential oil

2 tablespoons distilled water

SAFETY TIPS

✦ Do not use essential oils high in methyl salicylate, such as wintergreen or sweet birch, topically especially if you are currently taking anticoagulants. Essential oils high in methyl salicylate can make the effects of anticoagulants stronger, which could lead to bleeding and hemorrhaging.

✦ If you are on prescribed medications that are delivered via skin patches, do not use essential oils on the skin near, adjacent to, or under where conventional drug patches are placed. Many common components of essential oils have demonstrated the capacity to enhance drug absorption via the skin, which could lead to toxic outcomes in these instances.

✦ Do not use massage oils containing essential oils as intimate lubricants, as they may be irritating to sensitive membranes. In addition, avoid contact with latex condoms, as essential oils can impact their integrity.

✦ Standard dilutions for topical applications range from 2 to 2.5 percent (16 to 20 drops per ounce of carrier or base), maxing out at 5 percent (36 drops per ounce) for blends of short-term use on small areas of the skin. Consider dilutions of 1 percent for daily skin care blends.

BEST PRACTICES

✦ Most blends should be used within 3 to 6 months of blending to avoid adverse skin reactions that can take place as a result of oxidation of the essential oils.

✦ Store blends made with aloe vera or water in clear containers to keep an eye out for signs of clouding or mold—if encountered, discard the blend and start over.

✦ Have fun! Experiment! Enjoy the time you spend coming up with your own unique and supportive blends!

MY NOTES

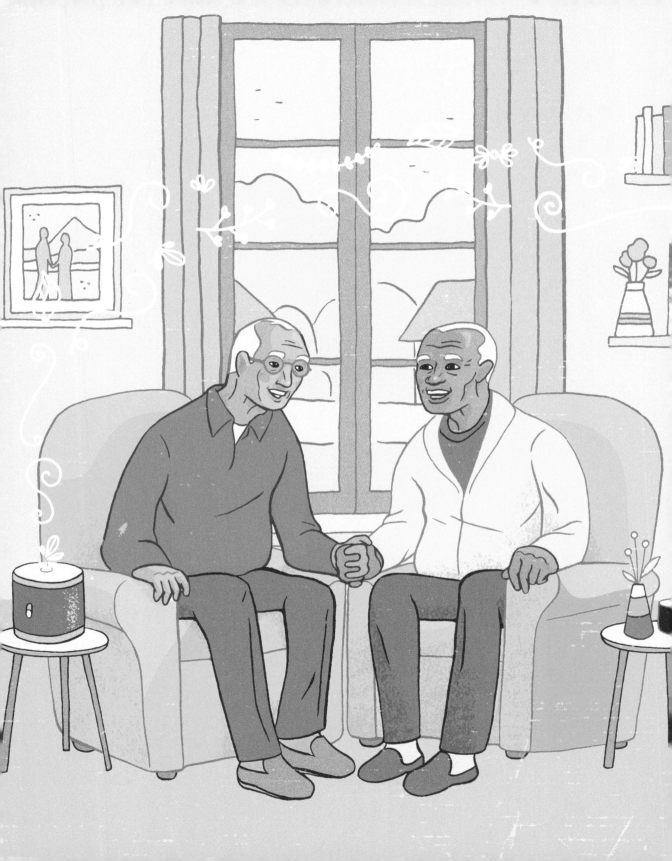

Chapter Six

SAFE BLENDS
FOR SENIORS

The Benefits of Aromatherapy as We Age

Becoming a senior in modern Western society is brimming with complex biological, social, economic, and emotional challenges. In a society that tends to place youth and vitality on an unsustainable pedestal, traversing this era of life may include the reality of being left behind, becoming isolated, and feeling undervalued.

As the physical body ages, there is increased likelihood of experiencing the adverse effects of the wear and tear accumulated over a lifetime's worth of experiences. The vitality governing our biological processes, such as healing and tissue repair, is not as sprightly as it once was, and illness, inflammation, and pain may be common. By the time people reach their mid-50s, there may also be multiple medications being consumed on a daily basis, some of which may produce disheartening side effects. Daily activities become more complicated to undertake as stiffness, balance, and wavering energy levels affect motivation and one's ability to get around. Sound sleep may be harder to achieve, and memory and cognition may become hazy, which can lead to increased tension, anxiety, and depression.

Time can take also take a toll on emotional and spiritual well-being, which may be the case if living in isolation from family members. Loneliness and feelings of disconnection can be common, especially as friends, partners, and loved ones are lost to long life. Retirement from a lifetime of work can also be unnerving; questions regarding one's identity and place in this world are coupled with the need to do something valuable and enjoyable with the time one has left. Chronic illness, expensive health care bills, making decisions about long-term care, and the loss of independence can all feed emotional distress and in turn create deeper imbalances in the physical body.

There is so much that aromatherapy can contribute to emotional and physical well-being, including supporting those with memory loss, agitation, grief, anxiety, and depression as well as those with loss of appetite, difficulty sleeping, balance problems, and joint pain and stiffness. In fact, most of the scientific research surrounding aromatherapy and seniors is focused on the use of essential oils as tools for compassionate care concerning wound healing, circulation, immunity, mobility, pain management, digestion, and rest and relaxation. Perhaps even more importantly, aromatherapy can reach beyond the provision of physical and emotional support by serving as a vehicle for connection and compassion, gifting empathy and empowerment to both the caregiver and care receiver. Whether a senior yourself or caring for seniors in your family, aromatherapy can be an incredible way to both stimulate and relax, soothe and motivate, and care and connect.

Safety Considerations for Essential Oils and Senior Citizens

There are a number of safety considerations for integrating essential oils into the lives of individuals over 55. Changes to the skin, the metabolism, and even the sense of smell can affect how sensitive aging individuals may be to essential oils. In addition, this age group is more likely to have multiple underlying health problems and use multiple prescription drugs, emphasizing the need for thoughtful essential oil choices. Lastly, if there are issues with cognition, memory, and physical or emotional discomfort, interacting with someone about essential oil preferences, gaining consent, and monitoring for adverse reactions may prove difficult. In this regard, it is important that the safe practice of aromatherapy also includes a cultivation of keen and compassionate awareness and respect.

Several changes take place in our skin as we age that dictate more careful consideration to the dosing of essential oils for topical use. These changes include reduced skin elasticity and thickness as well as a slowing of cellular turnover and repair. In this regard, the skin may be more prone to wounding and take much longer to heal. Age-related changes to the skin can also lead to an increased risk for sensitization or allergic reactions to essential oils, and skin that is wounded, diseased, or otherwise inflamed will be more sensitive, as well. In addition, if an individual is on prescription steroids or blood thinners, the skin can become quite fragile and can easily bruise, so when applying essential oil blends topically, you will need to remember to do so gently.

In addition to increased skin sensitivity, essential oil safety experts claim that seniors may be more easily systemically influenced by the potent nature of essential oils as a result of a general slowing of metabolism and elimination that takes place as we age. Within this context, a slowed metabolism manifests as a reduced capacity to process essential oil chemical components that come in contact with the skin and those that get absorbed into the bloodstream. Systemic sensitivity may also be more likely with people who are suffering with liver and/or kidney disease, as these are the two main organs involved in the metabolism and removal of foreign substances, like essential oils, from the body. Although it is unclear what types of adverse reactions may occur with the topical or aromatic use of essential oils as a result of a slowed metabolism, the general consensus is that lower doses of essential oils are needed to achieve wellness goals in this age group.

All of these factors combined have led essential oil safety experts to recommend more dilute topical applications of essential oils than you would use for younger adults. Although the general dilution for topical application of essential oils to adult skin runs between 2.5 percent and 5 percent, a 1 percent dilution (8 drops per ounce of carrier) is usually deemed appropriate for elders with sensitive skin; for daily skin care products, such as facial moisturizers; and when applying essential oils to large areas of an individual's body (for example, legs, arms, and back massage). Hydrosols can also be considered here for their gentle yet effective nature. Interestingly, several essential oil research studies looking into the effects of essential oils in supporting pain management and wound healing in seniors have used concentrations as high as 20 percent for small, local applications. However, 5 percent (36 drops per ounce) is likely as high as you would want to go for localized pain management or wound healing support without the guidance of a qualified health care professional.

Individuals over 55 may have several underlying health conditions that require the use of multiple medications, thus theoretically increasing the risk for essential oil interactions with pharmaceuticals. Although essential oil and drug interactions are unlikely with topical or aromatic use of essential oils (see Known Prescription Interactions, page 172), there have been several case reports that excessive topical use of certain essential oil components, such as methyl salicylate from wintergreen, alongside strong blood thinners may be problematic. Essential oils can also increase the absorption of pharmaceuticals through the skin and should therefore not be used under or adjacent to transdermal patches.

Lastly, there may be issues surrounding consent for aromatherapy with seniors who are suffering with memory loss from dementia or Alzheimer's disease or are otherwise incapacitated or nonverbal. It is always best practice not to force aromatherapy on someone who may not be able to consent to its use. In fact, keeping an individual's comfort in mind is of utmost importance, especially for those who are uncomfortable lying down or for those who are confined to a bed. Foot and hand massage and foot baths are often the easiest and most enjoyable methods of topical application, but diffusion, personal inhalers, and aromatherapy jewelry can be used in situations when there is a dislike of or lack of consent for any form of touch.

Respectful attention will also need to be paid to signs of adverse reactions, such as skin irritation, in those who are noncommunicative. In addition, many individuals will experience slight to significant loss in sense of smell as they age. It will be important to remember that an individual's inability to smell essential oils due to a loss of sense of smell does not mean that higher doses or more frequent use of essential oils is needed.

Comforting Connection Hand Massage Blend

CHILDREN 6+, TEENS, ADULTS, SENIORS

1% DILUTION

TO MAKE THE BLEND

Add the essential oils to a dark glass bottle with a dropper. Swirl the oils to blend. Add the sesame oil, cap the bottle tightly, and shake it well. Label and store the blend in a cool, dark place, and use it within 6 months of blending.

TO USE THE BLEND

Apply a few drops onto the back of the hands and gently massage wrists, back of hands, palms, and fingers, being mindful of painful or swollen joints. During acute bouts of anxiety, agitation, sundowning, or other challenging moments, have the individual bring the palms of their hands to their face and breathe deeply through their nose several times throughout the hand massage.

TIP: This blend can also be used on the feet. After a foot massage, be sure to clean feet of excess oil to reduce the chance of slipping and falling.

TOPICAL

MAKES 1 OUNCE

2 drops rose essential oil

3 drops ylang-ylang essential oil

3 drops sweet orange essential oil

2 tablespoons cold-pressed sesame oil or other light nut or seed oil

Energized and Motivated Personal Inhaler or Diffusion Blend

TO MAKE THE BLEND

Add the essential oils to a dark glass dropper bottle and swirl the oils to blend. Close the bottle tightly and be sure to label it. Store the blend in a cool, dark place, and use it within 6 months of blending.

TO USE THE BLEND

Apply 10 to 15 drops to the wick of an aromatherapy inhaler for use as needed. Similarly, 1 to 2 drops can be applied to aromatherapy jewelry, a cotton ball, or a facial tissue to carry around for use as needed. If using an aromatherapy diffuser, follow the manufacturer's instructions regarding the number of essential oil drops to use per diffusion. Diffuse for 30 to 60 minutes at a time one or two times a day.

TIP: This blend can also be used as an aromatherapy room mist. Add 15 to 30 drops to 1 ounce of distilled water in a glass bottle with an aromatizer. Spritz around a room as needed. Shake well before use.

AROMATIC

MAKES ½ OUNCE

1½ teaspoons sweet basil essential oil

1 teaspoon lemon essential oil

½ teaspoon sage essential oil

Live Spryly Joint Rub

2% DILUTION

TO MAKE THE RUB

Gently warm the coconut oil in a double boiler or bain-marie until it is soft enough to stir (aloe vera gel should not be heated). Remove the coconut oil from heat and allow it to cool until it's just warmer than body temperature (or it's just beginning to solidify). The coconut oil should be close to room temperature when adding essential oils. Add the essential oils to the coconut oil and stir until thoroughly blended. Scoop into a glass jar with a tight-fitting lid, and label it. Store the jar in a cool, dark place, and use it within 6 to 12 months of blending if using coconut oil, or 3 to 6 months if using aloe vera gel.

TO USE THE RUB

Apply to joints as needed up to three times a day. Make sure to wash hands after use. This blend is safe for daily use on small areas of the body.

TOPICAL

MAKES ABOUT 1 CUP

1 cup unrefined coconut oil (solid at room temperature) or aloe vera gel

40 drops frankincense essential oil or benzoin essential oil

40 drops peppermint essential oil

20 drops black pepper essential oil

20 drops clove essential oil

Lose the Bruise Salve

TO MAKE THE SALVE

Make sure to have a jar or salve tins ready. Heat the olive oil, herbal-infused oils, and beeswax in a double boiler or bain-marie until the beeswax is melted. Stir occasionally to ensure everything is well mixed. Remove from heat and allow to cool until just warmer than body temperature (or the mixture is just beginning to solidify). Add the essential oils and stir until they are thoroughly blended in with the oil and wax. Pour or spoon the salve into the prepared container(s). Label and store the jar in a cool, dark location. Use it within 6 to 12 months of blending.

TO USE THE SALVE

Using clean fingers or a cotton swab, apply a pea-sized or smaller amount of salve to the bruised area, gently rubbing into the area until absorbed. This salve can be used safely on a daily basis as needed up to three times a day.

TIP: Use a bit more beeswax for a harder salve and less beeswax for a softer salve. Avoid adding essential oils to a really hot oil-wax blend as they can evaporate and oxidize, which compromises the quality of your salve.

TOPICAL

MAKES 1½ CUPS

¼ cup cold-pressed olive oil

½ cup arnica herbal-infused oil (*not* essential oil)

½ cup St. John's wort herbal-infused oil

¼ cup beeswax beads or shavings

30 drops helichrysum essential oil

30 drops yarrow essential oil

20 drops rosemary essential oil

15 drops black pepper essential oil

Brain Food Concentration and Memory Support Personal Roll-On

CHILDREN 12+, TEENS, ADULTS, SENIORS

2% DILUTION

TO MAKE THE BLEND

Add the essential oils to a roller bottle and gently swirl the oils to mix. Fill the bottle to the top with the fractionated coconut oil. Close it with the rollerball and cap, and shake it to combine. Label and store the bottle in a cool dark location. Use it within 6 months of blending.

TO USE THE BLEND

Gently dab on the temples and massage them as needed. You can also use it on the inner wrists and behind the ears as needed to support concentration and memory recall.

TOPICAL, AROMATIC

MAKES ½ OUNCE

4 drops rosemary essential oil

2 drops sweet basil essential oil

2 drops bay laurel essential oil

1 tablespoon fractionated coconut oil or cold-pressed sesame oil

A Healthy Dose of Hungry Diffusion Blend for Appetite Support

CHILDREN 12+, TEENS, ADULTS, SENIORS

TO MAKE THE BLEND

Add the essential oils to a dark glass dropper bottle and swirl the oils to blend. Cap the bottle tightly and don't forget to label the blend. Store it in a cool, dark location, and use it within 6 months of blending.

TO USE THE BLEND

Follow the manufacturer's instructions regarding the number of essential oil drops to use in the diffuser. Diffuse for 20 to 30 minutes before mealtimes. Alternatively, add 15 to 30 drops of the blend and 1 ounce of distilled water to a glass bottle with an aromatizer to use as an aromatherapy mist, shaking well before use.

AROMATIC

MAKES ½ OUNCE

1½ teaspoons lemon essential oil

1 teaspoon cardamom essential oil

½ teaspoon ginger essential oil

Hard to Heal Wound Support First Aid Mist

CHILDREN 12+, TEENS, ADULTS, SENIORS

5% DILUTION

TO MAKE THE CLEANSING MIST

Add the essential oils to a 2-ounce dark glass bottle with an aromatizer. Swirl the oils to blend. Add the vegetable glycerin and lavender hydrosol to the bottle, cap it tightly, and shake vigorously. Label and store the mist in a cool, dark place. Use it within 3 to 6 months of blending.

TO USE THE CLEANSING MIST

Shake very well before use. Apply a few spritzes to a clean wound before dressing with a bandage. If irritation or stinging occurs, discontinue use or consider using a more diluted blend (1 to 2 percent instead of 5 percent). At a 5 percent dilution, this mist is meant to be used only on small, localized areas of the body. Avoid contact with the face and sensitive membranes.

TIP: This mist can be used in conjunction with other wound-dressing protocols. However, please speak to your doctor or other health care provider before using it on chronic wounds, such as diabetic ulcers and bedsores.

TOPICAL

MAKES ABOUT 2 OUNCES

20 drops tea tree
   essential oil
20 drops yarrow essential oil
20 drops helichrysum
   essential oil
12 drops German chamomile
   essential oil
1 tablespoon vegetable
   glycerin
3 tablespoons lavender
   hydrosol

Go with the Flow Relieving Foot Bath

TEENS, ADULTS
1% DILUTION

TO MAKE THE SOAKING SALT

Combine all the essential oils in a glass measuring cup. Add the olive oil and mix well. Add the Epsom salt and mix together. Spoon the mixture into a glass jar with a tight-fitting lid. Label and store the soaking salt in a cool, dark place. Use it within 6 months of blending.

TO USE THE SOAKING SALT

Add ⅛ cup of the soaking salt to warm water in a vessel large enough for at least one foot. Soak feet for 10 to 15 minutes to support healthy circulation and joint mobility.

TIP: Follow up a footbath with gentle foot and leg massage using Maintain the Flow Circulation Support Massage Blend (see below).

TOPICAL

MAKES ABOUT ½ CUP

10 drops frankincense essential oil
10 drops vetiver essential oil
12 drops cypress essential oil
1 tablespoon cold-pressed olive oil or calendula herbal-infused oil
½ cup Epsom salt

Maintain the Flow Circulation Support Massage Blend

TEENS, ADULTS
1% DILUTION

TO MAKE THE BLEND

Add the essential oils to a dark glass bottle with a dropper. Swirl the oils to blend. Add the olive oil, cap it tightly, and shake the bottle vigorously until blended. Label and store the blend in a cool, dark place. Use it within 6 months of blending.

TO USE THE BLEND

Using this blend is easier with two people, a giver and a receiver. Warm a few drops in your hands and elevate the receiver's feet to a comfortable level, preferably above the heart. Gently massage the feet and lower legs using light stroking movements toward the heart. Avoid direct pressure on wounds, varicose veins, and bruises.

TOPICAL

MAKES 1 OUNCE

4 drops rosemary essential oil
2 drops cypress essential oil
2 drops cedarwood essential oil
2 tablespoons cold-pressed olive oil

Off to Neverland Sleep Support Diffusion or Room Mist Blend

CHILDREN 12+, TEENS, ADULTS, SENIORS

TO MAKE THE BLEND

Add the essential oils to a small, dark glass dropper bottle and swirl the oils to blend. Cap the bottle tightly and don't forget to label the blend. Store it in a cool, dark location, and use it within 6 months of blending.

TO USE THE BLEND

Follow the manufacturer's instructions regarding the number of essential oil drops to use in the diffuser. Diffuse for 20 to 30 minutes before bed. Alternatively, add 15 to 30 drops of the blend and 1 ounce of distilled water to a glass bottle with an aromatizer to use as an aromatherapy mist, shaking well before use. This mist can also be sprayed on bed linens and pillows.

AROMATIC

MAKES ½ OUNCE

1½ teaspoons clary sage essential oil

1 teaspoon ylang-ylang essential oil

½ teaspoon hops essential oil

Respiratory and Immune Support Diffusion or Personal Inhaler Blend

CHILDREN 12+, TEENS, ADULTS, SENIORS

TO MAKE THE BLEND

Add the essential oils to a small, dark glass dropper bottle and swirl the oils to mix. Cap the bottle tightly and label the blend. Store it in a cool, dark place, and use it within 6 months of blending.

TO USE THE BLEND

Follow the manufacturer's instructions regarding the number of essential oil drops to use in the diffuser. Diffuse for 30 to 60 minutes up to three times daily for immune and breathing support. Alternatively, apply 10 to 15 drops to the wick of an aromatherapy inhaler and use as needed, or apply 1 to 2 drops to aromatherapy jewelry, a cotton ball, or a facial tissue to carry with you to use as needed.

AROMATIC

MAKES ½ OUNCE

1 teaspoon eucalyptus essential oil

1 teaspoon benzoin essential oil

½ teaspoon myrtle essential oil

½ teaspoon thyme essential oil

SAFETY TIPS

❖ Remember that thin, abraded, or inflamed skin may be more sensitive to irritation from essential oils. When in doubt, use a patch test for any oils you may be concerned about.

❖ The dose of essential oils being used with individuals over 55 may need to be lower than that for robust, younger adults, certainly if there is sensitivity of the skin, multiple underlying health problems and/or pharmaceutical medications, and/or a compromised immune system. When blending essential oils for seniors, you will need to consider their general constitution and health status for dilution ratios.

❖ One percent dilution is considered standard for this age group for cosmetic applications and topical use on large areas of the body. However, depending on the nature of an individual's constitution and health status, 2.5 percent to 5 percent dilution for topical applications may also be considered safe, especially when applied for short periods of time on small, localized areas of the body.

❖ The risk of interactions between drugs and essential oils is minimal with topical or aromatic oil use but potentially significant with internal or oral oil use. When in doubt, speak to your doctor prior to trying anything new, especially if you are taking blood thinners. Please refer to chapter 5 (see page 79) and Known Prescription Interactions (see page 172) for drug interaction considerations.

BEST PRACTICES

- Ensure you are receiving consent before using essential oils on or around seniors. Do not force aromatherapy or essential oils on anyone who is refusing them, even if you think it is in their best interest. Aroma can become powerfully imprinted in memories, and aromatherapy is meant to be a relaxing and supportive modality.

- Even if an individual cannot smell essential oils strongly due to a loss of sense of smell, a higher dose or more frequent use of essential oils is not needed. Stick with safe dilution and diffusion protocols, and trust that the essential oils are doing their work even if they can't be smelled.

- Respectful attention will need to be paid to signs of adverse reactions, such as skin irritation, in those who are noncommunicative or otherwise incapacitated. Use patch testing on thin, sensitive skin before using a new essential oil over large areas of the body.

MY NOTES

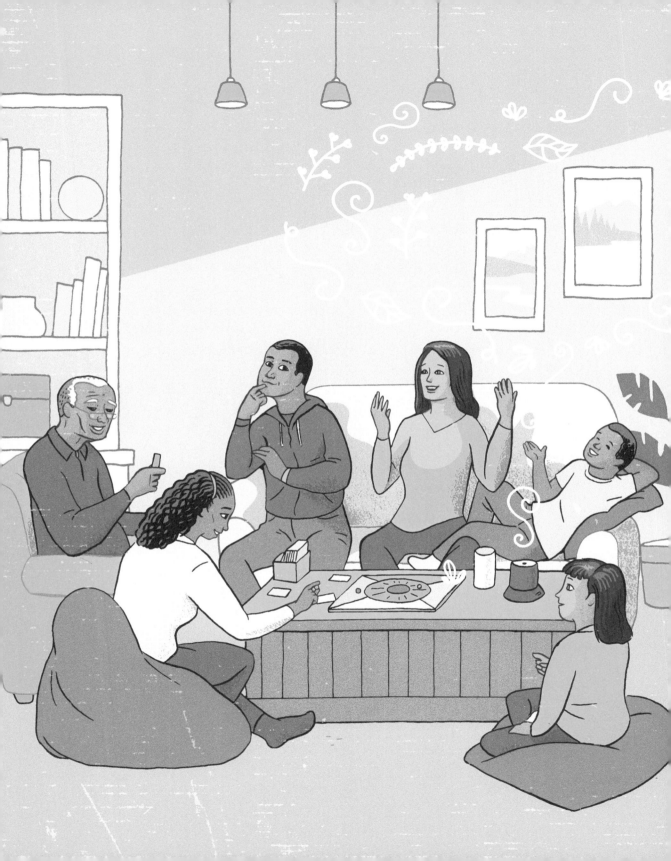

Chapter Seven

BLENDS FOR
YOUR HOUSEHOLD

Benefits of Aromatherapy in the Household

Beyond supporting the physical and emotional needs of your family, essential oils can serve as safe and enjoyable alternatives to regular household cleaning products and washing detergents, many of which are rife with harsh chemicals. In addition, "superbugs," including species of yeast and bacteria, have begun to build resistance to these chemicals, and there is a growing belief among health professionals that the sterile environments created by these products also contribute to a lack of human resistance to infection.

Not only do essential oils smell lovely and provide wonderful aromatic support for our minds and bodies, they are also disinfecting antimicrobial powerhouses that can be used safely and effectively in maintaining a fresh and clean home without stripping your household environment of its own innate defenses or causing toxic reactions in your body or the bodies of your loved ones. Essential oils are also great for cutting through grease and grime from dishes and sticky surfaces as well as repelling household pests, such as moths, pavement ants, rodents, and cockroaches. Lastly, making your own "green cleaning" products can be a creative and fun family activity as long as safety is paramount.

Safety Considerations for Household Blends

Choosing which essential oils to use to clean and freshen up your home requires special considerations. Firstly, you may want to reserve expensive oils, such as rose, neroli, or jasmine, for topical or aromatic use. It is also advised to refrain from using hard-to-find essential oils or oils distilled from endangered plants. Indeed, it is important to consider whether or not it is a holistic, environmentally friendly practice to use essential oils from threatened or endangered species in any of your aromatherapy blends.

Essential oils expressed from the peels of citrus species, such as sweet orange, lemon, and grapefruit, are often a by-product of the food and beverage industry and in many ways represent the most sustainable option for making household cleaners. In addition, these essential oils have a very short shelf life, averaging about six months, when they become oxidized and are no longer therapeutically useful. However, instead of throwing these essential oils away, you can use them in your green cleaning products. The same goes for any essential oils that have been sitting on your shelf for too long and may no longer be entirely trustworthy for their therapeutic effects. Rather than throwing oils away, throw them in your cleaning supplies instead.

A second consideration for choosing which essential oils to use in your household cleaning and washing blends surrounds which oils are deemed safe for all members of your family, including pets. For example, if you have infants or young children in your family, you may want to consider washing clothing and linens only with essential oils deemed safe for these age groups. There is general consensus within the aromatherapy community that using essential oils for cleaning products provides a little more leeway in this regard. For example, although white pine essential oil is not considered safe for infants for topical or aromatic use, it may be just fine to blend it into cleaning products used on bathroom or kitchen surfaces as long as it does not come in direct contact with your infant's skin and your infant is not unnecessarily overexposed to the aroma of these products.

Using essential oils to clean toys or other objects that may be placed in a baby's or child's mouth is not advisable. In these instances, hot water and soap may be all that is required. Also be mindful of exposure to surfaces that have recently been cleaned with sprays or scrubs containing essential oils. Just like bleach or ammonia, you will not want residues of these products coming into contact with anyone's skin, especially if using essential oils that are old and have oxidized, making them even more irritating to the skin. In this regard, just like with traditional household cleaners, gloves should be worn when using cleaning products with essential oils. Make sure to wash your hands, and the hands of your helpers, after blending or using green cleaning and washing products made with essential oils.

It is important to note that essential oils considered safe for humans may actually be toxic to your pets. As beloved members of your family, you will want to keep pet safety in mind as you use essential oils around your home. The bodies of household pets, such as cats and dogs, have different physiology than human beings, including varying capacities to process and detoxify chemicals from essential oils. Whereas an essential oil may be non-toxic to a human, a cat or a dog could experience significant or life-threatening adverse reactions. Much like infants and young children, pets may be unable to get away from strong smells that are irritating or toxic to them, especially if they are enclosed in cages or behind closed doors. If using essential oils in a home with pets, it is best practice to make sure that they are able to leave a room, go outside, or otherwise have access to fresh air. Also, refrain from using essential oils, either diluted or undiluted, on objects or surfaces that may facilitate direct contact or ingestion of the essential oils by your pets. These objects include but are not limited to litter boxes, food and water bowls, pet toys, and pet beds. Lastly, although there are a variety of uses for essential oils for cats and dogs, it is critical that you speak to your veterinarian prior to using essential oils with your pets in order to avoid serious and life-threatening outcomes.

First Aid for Essential Oil Exposure

If the safety protocols that are outlined in each chapter of this book have been followed, adverse reactions to essential oils are unlikely to be common. However, accidental over-exposure or ingestion can take place and lead to severe and sometimes life-threatening outcomes. In order to ensure essential oils are being safely integrated into your home, it is a good idea to become familiar with some standard first aid procedures in the likelihood of adverse reactions following exposure to essential oils. The following is adapted from *Essential Oil Safety (2nd edition)*, by Robert Tisserand and Rodney Young.

Ingestion: If you believe essential oils have been ingested accidentally, do not induce vomiting, which can further damage sensitive mucous membranes of the stomach, esophagus, and mouth. Vomiting can also lead to aspiration or the intake of vomit and essential oils into the lungs. If the person is conscious, you can attempt to rinse their mouth with water. In all cases, you should immediately head to the nearest hospital. *Do not forget to take the bottle with you.* You may also want to call poison control and follow the agency's instructions.

Inhalation: If you suspect an adverse reaction is taking place in response to the aromatic use of essential oils, immediately remove the person or pet to fresh air and seek medical attention.

Eye contact: If either diluted or undiluted essential oils come in direct contact with eyes, flush the eyes with vegetable oil for 15 minutes, and follow with a water or saline rinse. If the person wears contact lenses, make sure the lenses are removed prior to flushing. Use a first aid eye cup for flushing to ensure proper rinsing. Seek medical attention if irritation occurs or persists.

Skin contact: Gently wash the skin with unscented liquid soap and warm water repeatedly for 15 minutes. Keep skin exposed to air (but not direct sunlight) to encourage evaporation of essential oils. If reactions are taking place over large areas of the skin, lukewarm baths with oatmeal can be soothing. If irritation persists or worsens, seek medical attention, especially for children under 12 years old, the elderly, or those who are ill or immune compromised.

ESSENTIAL OIL SUSTAINABILITY

Essential oils require a huge volume of natural resources to produce. Hundreds of pounds of plant material are needed for just one gallon of essential oil, and this ratio changes depending on the species of plant being distilled. Some plants yield less essential oil than others, requiring even more plant material to procure the same amount of essential oil as a higher-yielding species.

Regardless of the species, the amount of plant material needed is very large, especially from plants that are harvested from the wild. If the plants are grown agriculturally, the amount of land, water, human labor, and fossil fuels needed to grow and harvest the thousands of pounds of plant material required to produce essential oils is immense.

In our attempts to create a more environmentally conscious and safe household, we must consider where our essential oils are coming from, how they are produced, their carbon footprint, and the impact their production has on natural resources, such as land, water, and fossil fuels. Keeping sustainability in the forefront of our minds, we can ensure that we are using these resource-heavy products prudently and with respect for the greater sociocultural and environmental impact of their production.

LIST OF ESSENTIAL OILS GREAT FOR HOUSEHOLD CLEANING PRODUCTS AND DETERGENTS

+ Clove
+ Grapefruit
+ Lavender
+ Lemon
+ Lemongrass
+ Sweet orange
+ Tea tree
+ Thyme
+ White pine

Household Blends

Quick and Easy Cleaning Wipes

KEEP OUT OF THE REACH OF CHILDREN

Add a few drops of essential oil directly onto a damp cleaning towel to wipe down and disinfect surfaces.

TIP: Do not use essential oils directly on furniture or finished surfaces, as some essential oils can strip them of their coatings/finishes. These cleaning wipes can also be incorporated into your floor-cleaning routines.

CLEANING

MAKES 1 CLEANING WIPE

3 to 5 drops lemongrass essential oil or white pine essential oil

Surface Spray for Mold and Disinfection

KEEP OUT OF THE REACH OF CHILDREN

1. Combine all the ingredients in a glass spray bottle, close it tightly, and shake well. Label and store the bottle in a cool, dark place away from the reach of children. Can be stored indefinitely.

2. Shake well before using. Spray surfaces and wipe down as normal. For extra mold-busting power, spray heavily and let sit for 12 to 24 hours before wiping down with warm water.

CLEANING

MAKES ABOUT 1 CUP

¾ cup distilled water
¼ cup isopropyl alcohol
1 or 2 drops unscented, biodegradable dish soap
15 drops lemongrass essential oil
15 drops tea tree essential oil
15 drops thyme essential oil

Surface Scrub for Deep Cleaning Grime and Grout

KEEP OUT OF THE REACH OF CHILDREN

1. Add the baking soda to a small mixing bowl. Slowly add water while stirring until a thick paste forms.

2. Add the essential oils and stir the paste thoroughly to ensure proper mixing of essential oils.

3. Apply to grimy surfaces, grout, or places that need a bit of abrasion for cleaning. Scrub vigorously and let sit for several minutes before wiping clean with warm water.

CLEANING

MAKES ½ CUP

½ cup baking soda
Water
5 drops tea tree essential oil
5 drops grapefruit
   essential oil

TIP: This cleaning scrub is best if made fresh each time you want to use it.

Sweet-Scented Laundry Detergent

KEEP OUT OF THE REACH OF CHILDREN

1. Combine all ingredients in a mixing bowl and mix well.

2. Transfer the mixture to a food processor and purée with a regular blade until powdery.

3. Transfer the detergent to a large glass jar with a tight-fitting lid, and label. Can be stored indefinitely.

4. To use the detergent, add 2 tablespoons to your washing machine's soap compartment for powder detergent.

TIP: Play around with the amount of detergent you use for each load. Depending on your washing machine design, you may want to use more or less than what is recommended here.

CLEANING

MAKES ABOUT 4 CUPS

1½ cups grated castile soap
1 cup borax
1 cup washing soda
½ cup baking soda
20 drops sweet orange
   essential oil
20 drops lavender
   essential oil

Mild Mannered Dishwashing Soap

CHILDREN 2+, TEENS, ADULTS, SENIORS

1. Combine all the ingredients in a quart-size canning jar or bottle with a pump top. Cap the bottle tightly and shake it vigorously to mix. Don't forget to label the soap.

2. Use 1 to 2 tablespoons in a sink full of warm water to wash or prewash dishes. Remember to use gloves as warm water may increase the possibility of skin irritation or sensitization.

TIP: Using water in this recipe is optional. However, it does make for easier blending and mixing with the essential oils. If you find this mixture to be too runny, omit the water from the recipe and reduce the essential oils to 40 drops of each.

CLEANING

MAKES 3 TO 4 CUPS

3 cups liquid castile soap or unscented, biodegradable dish soap
1 cup water (optional)
50 drops lemon essential oil
50 drops lavender essential oil

Mothballs for Drawers and Closets

KEEP OUT OF THE REACH OF CHILDREN

1. Combine the essential oils in a small bowl and mix well.

2. Using a glass dropper or pipette, add 2 drops of the blend to each cotton ball.

3. Place 1 or 2 cotton balls in a nylon stocking and hang in your closet, and place the remaining balls in your drawers, to deter moths and silverfish.

4. Keep the mothballs away from the reach of children and pets. Replace as needed, or about once a month.

HOUSEHOLD

MAKES 6 BALLS

6 drops lavender essential oil
6 drops clove essential oil
6 organic cotton balls

Concentrated Floor-Cleaning Solution

1. Combine all the ingredients in a glass measuring cup. Using a fork, stir vigorously until mixed.

2. Pour into a glass canning jar. Cover the opening of the jar with wax paper before screwing on the lid. The wax paper creates a barrier between the vinegar and the metal of the lid so the lid won't rust. After screwing on the lid, label and store in cool, dark place. This blend can be stored indefinitely. Add more essential oils over time if the scent begins to fade.

3. To use the floor cleaner, shake vigorously and pour a small amount into a mop bucket. Fill the bucket with hot water. Mop floors as usual.

TIP: Avoid using on finished wood floors, as the solution might remove the finish. Also not recommended to use on stone floors due to the presence of white vinegar. It is always best practice to do a test patch in a small area that won't be seen to ensure that you won't damage your floors (think about it like a patch test on people). Safe for use on linoleum and tile but might be damaging to laminate flooring. Test first.

CLEANING

MAKES ABOUT 1½ CUPS

½ cup isopropyl alcohol

½ cup white vinegar

½ cup unscented, biodegradable dish soap

1 tablespoon olive oil or similar oil

20 drops white pine essential oil

20 drops lemon essential oil

10 drops thyme essential oil

Carpet Deodorizing Powder

CLEANING

MAKES 2 CUPS

1½ cups baking soda
½ cup kaolin clay
20 drops sweet orange
  essential oil
15 drops lavender
  essential oil
15 drops lemongrass
  essential oil
10 drops thyme essential oil

1. Combine the baking soda and kaolin clay in a bowl and mix well.

2. In a separate bowl, combine the essential oils and stir to blend.

3. Using a fork or whisk to stir, slowly add the essential oils to the powder. Stir well until completely blended, breaking up any clumps that are created when adding the essential oils.

4. Transfer the powder to a glass canning jar with a tight-fitting lid for use and storage. Do not forget to label. This powder can be kept indefinitely. Add more essential oils if it begins to lose its scent.

5. Vacuum your carpet to remove debris, pet hair, dust, and dirt before using the powder. Lightly sprinkle powder on the carpet and let it sit undisturbed for 10 to 15 minutes before vacuuming. You may need to vacuum twice before the powder is fully removed from the carpet. Make sure that children and pets do not come in contact with the powder, and consider not allowing children or pets on the newly deodorized carpet for at least an hour after use, to ensure that any irritating essential oils do not come in contact with their skin.

TIP: Consider using a glass dropper to add the essential oils to the powder while mixing rather than pouring them in. This method can make for overall smooth and thorough blending. If you would like to be able to sprinkle powder on carpets more easily, consider poking several small holes into a piece of aluminum foil large enough to cover the opening of the canning jar. Use the ring of the canning jar lid to secure the aluminum foil in place while shaking powder on carpet. When finished using, replace the aluminum foil with the proper lid for storage.

SAFETY TIPS

- Always wear gloves when making or using cleaning and washing products made with essential oils.

- Label all your cleaning and washing products well, and consider storing them separately from aromatherapy blends that are being used topically or aromatically in order to avoid confusion.

- When blending essential oils for clothing, towel, diaper, and bed linen washing products, blend with the youngest members of your family in mind, and use only essential oils deemed safe for that age group.

- Keep all essential oils and aromatherapy blends and products away from the reach of children and pets.

- Refrain from using essential oils, either diluted or undiluted, on objects or surfaces that may facilitate direct contact or ingestion of essential oils by young children or pets. Do not use essential oils to clean toys that can end up in a child's mouth.

- If using cleaning or washing products in a home with pets, make sure that pets have access to fresh air, and avoid using those products in ways that will directly expose your pets' skin or mouths.

- Follow first aid safety procedures if accidental ingestion, exposure, or adverse reactions take place. If seeking medical attention, don't forget to take the essential oil bottle with you.

BEST PRACTICES

- Avoid using essential oils on finished wood floors, as the oils might remove the finish. It is always best practice to do a test patch in a small area that won't be seen to ensure that you won't damage your floors (think about it like a patch test on people).

- Don't use essential oils directly on furniture, as they can strip surfaces.

- Cleaning products made with vinegar may not be appropriate for stone surfaces or grout applications.

- If essential oils become too old or oxidized for topical or aromatic use, don't throw them away. Instead, consider using them in cleaning and washing products, saving your new, therapeutically potent essential oils for topical or aromatic use.

- Keep sustainability in the forefront of your mind when using essential oils in your home and with your family. Use essential oils prudently and respectfully, and take breaks from time to time. Also, never use essential oils produced from threatened or endangered species.

MY NOTES

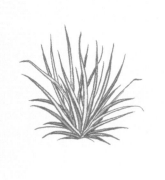
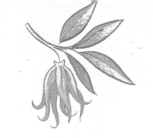
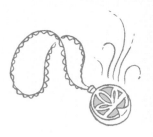
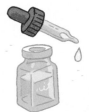
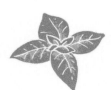
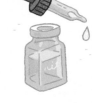
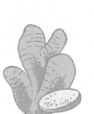

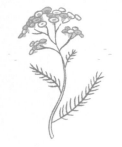
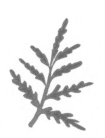
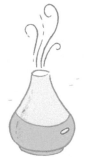
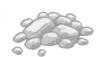
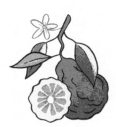
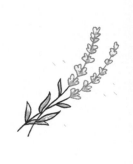

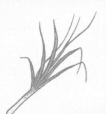
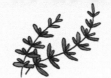
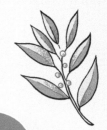
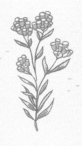
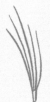
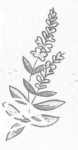

Part II

30 FAMILY-FRIENDLY ESSENTIAL OILS TO KNOW

Part II of this book is dedicated to 30 essential oils that can be safely and enjoyably integrated into your home and the lives of your family members. The essential oils in this section appear in recipes throughout this book and have been chosen for their versatility, sustainability, and safety profiles as well as their cost-effectiveness. For a more detailed description of uses and recipes, please refer to the Ailments and Oils Quick-Reference Guide (page 160) and chapters within this book.

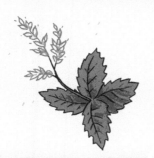

Chapter Eight

TOP 30 SAFE OILS

Bay Laurel

Laurus nobilis

SPICY, SWEET SCENT

COST: $

Also known as sweet bay or laurel leaf, bay laurel essential oil offers an uplifting fragrance, with hints of camphor and spice. Sourced from the same plant as bay leaves used for culinary purposes, this essential oil is ideal for diffusing when you have a cold or the flu. You can also diffuse it when you're feeling stressed and on the edge of illness; it supports a healthy immune system and promotes clarity and peace of mind.

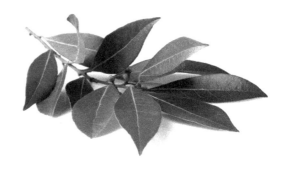

MEDICINAL PROPERTIES
Analgesic, antibacterial, antiseptic, antispasmodic, antiviral, astringent, cholagogue, emmenagogue, expectorant, febrifuge, insecticide, sedative, stomachic, sudorific

USED FOR
Cold and flu; ideal for supporting digestive health

BLENDS WELL WITH
Bergamot, clary sage, cypress, eucalyptus, frankincense, ginger, juniper berry, lavender, lemon, myrtle, patchouli, pine, Ravensara leaf, ravintsara, rosemary, Spanish sage, sweet orange, ylang-ylang

PRECAUTIONS
Do not use during pregnancy. Bay laurel can cause skin irritation.

Benzoin

Styrax benzoin, S. tonkinensis

WARM, SWEET SCENT

COST: $$

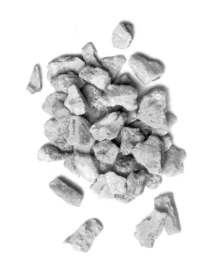

With a pleasant aroma that carries a strong hint of vanilla, benzoin essential oil is very popular with perfumeries and incense makers. Historically used in India and Asia, it was also quite popular with ancient Egyptians. It is no surprise, then, that this beautiful oil is ideal for alleviating stress and creating a sense of euphoria.

MEDICINAL PROPERTIES
Antidepressant, anti-inflammatory, antiseptic, astringent, carminative, cordial, deodorant, diuretic, expectorant, sedative, vulnerary

USED FOR
Arthritis, rheumatism, body aches, and joint pains; ideal for relieving chapped, dry skin

BLENDS WELL WITH
Bergamot, black pepper, cinnamon leaf, coriander, cypress, frankincense, ginger, jasmine, juniper berry, lavender, lemon, marjoram, myrrh, petitgrain, rose, rosemary, sandalwood, sweet orange

PRECAUTIONS
Avoid use before driving or undertaking important tasks.

Bergamot

Citrus bergamia

SPICY, CITRUS SCENT

COST: $$

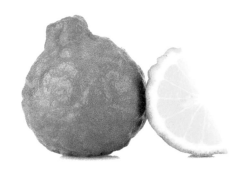

A valuable essential oil for helping with oily skin, abscesses, and boils, bergamot is also a good choice for dealing with stress and exhaustion. If you suffer from seasonal depression, you may find that diffusing bergamot is a good way to lift your mood and give you the inspiration you need to get up and go. Choose bergamot FCF, which stands for "furocoumarin free," if possible; it has had the bergapten (furocoumarin) removed and is far less phototoxic than standard bergamot.

MEDICINAL PROPERTIES

Analgesic, antidepressant, antiseptic, antispasmodic, calmative, cicatrizant, deodorant, digestive, febrifuge, stomachic, vermifuge, vulnerary

USED FOR

Acne, oily skin, psoriasis, and eczema; ideal for making bath and body products

BLENDS WELL WITH

Basil, clary sage, coriander, cypress, geranium, German chamomile, ginger, hops flower, jasmine, juniper berry, palo santo, Roman chamomile, rose, sandalwood, vetiver

PRECAUTIONS

Phototoxic if not labeled "bergamot FCF"; do not apply to skin that will be exposed to direct sunlight. Bergamot can cause sensitive skin.

Black Pepper

Piper nigrum

WARM, SPICY SCENT

COST: $

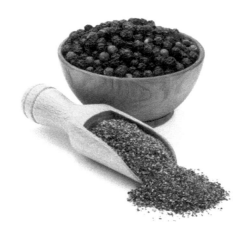

Offering a crisp, spicy scent with hints of green and the slightest touch of flowers, black pepper essential oil smells a little bit like freshly ground peppercorns. It stimulates the mind and promotes alertness. Its ability to facilitate circulation while providing a deep, warming effect makes it a good choice in blends designed to ease muscle pain and aching joints.

MEDICINAL PROPERTIES

Analgesic, antiseptic, antispasmodic, aphrodisiac, diaphoretic, digestive, diuretic, febrifuge, laxative, rubefacient

USED FOR

Digestive problems, arthritis, flu, and cold; ideal for use in blends designed to provide emotional motivation

BLENDS WELL WITH

Bergamot, clary sage, clove bud, coriander, fennel seed, frankincense, geranium, ginger, grapefruit, juniper berry, lavender, lemon, lime, mandarin, sandalwood, Spanish sage, rosewood, ylang-ylang

PRECAUTIONS

Avoid topical use during pregnancy due to increased risk of skin sensitization. Black pepper can cause sensitive skin.

Blue Gum Eucalyptus

Eucalyptus globulus

MINTY SCENT

COST: $

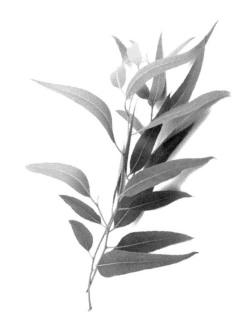

Also known as Tasmanian blue gum or Southern blue gum, the evergreen tree this oil comes from is widely cultivated in places such as Australia, Africa, and New Zealand and often serves as both a home and food source to koala bears. The infamous minty oil of this tree's leaves is steam distilled and is believed to improve respiratory conditions as it provides antioxidant protection, aids in circulation, and stimulates the immune system.

MEDICINAL PROPERTIES
Analgesic, antibacterial, anti-inflammatory, antimalarial, antimicrobial, antipyretic, antirheumatic, antiseborrheic, antiseptic, antispasmodic, decongestant, diuretic, expectorant, stimulant

USED FOR
Bronchitis, COPD, and pneumonia; ideal for helping ailments that involve difficulties breathing

BLENDS WELL WITH
Basil, cedarwood, frankincense, ginger, lavender, lemon, myrtle, tea tree

PRECAUTIONS
Do not use during pregnancy or breast-feeding or with young children.

Cedarwood

Juniperus virginiana

SOFT, WOODY SCENT

COST: $

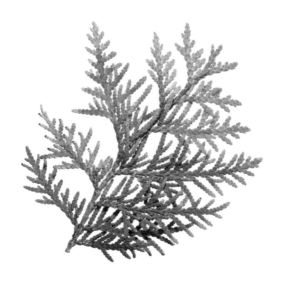

Sometimes confused with Atlas cedarwood, this essential oil comes from Virginian red cedar trees, which are also known as eastern red, Bedford, or southern red cedars. Prized by Native Americans, the oldest examples of these trees are estimated to have sprouted over 900 years ago. Like many other products made with this beautiful red wood, cedarwood essential oil deters insect activity. Its soft fragrance helps soothe nervous tension and ease anxiety.

MEDICINAL PROPERTIES
Antiseborrheic, antiseptic, antispasmodic, astringent, diuretic, emmenagogue, expectorant, fungicide, insect repellent, insecticide, sedative

USED FOR
Arthritis, respiratory illnesses, and urinary tract infections; ideal for making products to combat oily skin and hair

BLENDS WELL WITH
Benzoin, bergamot, cinnamon leaf, citronella, cypress, frankincense, helichrysum, jasmine, juniper berry, lavender, lemon, lime, neroli, rose, rose geranium, rosemary

PRECAUTIONS
Do not use during pregnancy. Cedarwood can cause skin irritation when used at high concentrations.

Clary Sage

Salvia sclarea

HERBACEOUS,
SLIGHTLY FRUITY SCENT

COST: $$

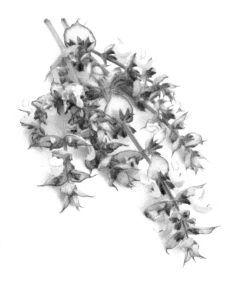

Clary sage is an excellent essential oil for relaxation, and when used in bedtime blends, it can lull you gently to sleep. It is most popular, though, for its value in alleviating PMS, painful periods, and menopause symptoms. It contains sclareol, a constituent with an estrogen-like structure that helps bring hormones into balance. When diffused or worn in personal fragrance blends, clary sage can promote a calm feeling of self-confidence.

MEDICINAL PROPERTIES

Antidepressant, anti-inflammatory, antiseptic, antispasmodic, aphrodisiac, astringent, bactericidal, carminative, deodorant, digestive, emmenagogue, euphoric, hypotensive, nervine, parturient, sedative, stomachic

USED FOR

Depression and postnatal depression; ideal for making relaxing bath and body products

BLENDS WELL WITH

Bergamot, cedarwood, frankincense, geranium, juniper berry, lavender, lemon, sandalwood, sweet orange, vitex berry

PRECAUTIONS

Do not use during pregnancy. Do not use before driving or operating machinery.

Cypress

Cupressus sempervirens

WOODY, SLIGHTLY SPICY SCENT

COST: $

Besides offering a very versatile essential oil, cypress has a fascinating history. Thanks to the wood's durability and resilience, it was used to carve Egyptian sarcophagi, and ancient Greeks often used it to carve statues of their gods. Because of its association with cemeteries and grave goods, cypress is nicknamed the "tree of death," but its botanical name alludes to its long life. Cypress essential oil has a long litany of uses, benefiting ailments as varied as hemorrhoids, muscle cramps, and stress.

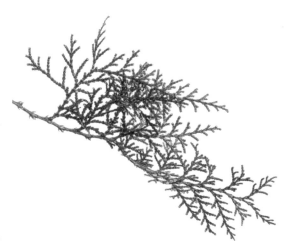

MEDICINAL PROPERTIES

Antiseptic, antispasmodic, astringent, calmative, deodorant, diuretic, hemostatic, hepatic, insect repellent, insecticide, sedative, styptic, sudorific, vasoconstrictor

USED FOR

Varicose veins, asthma, bronchitis, and flu; ideal for making massage blends for muscle aches and cramping

BLENDS WELL WITH

Bergamot, clary sage, copaiba, frankincense, helichrysum, juniper berry, lavender, marjoram, myrtle, pine, Ravensara leaf, rosemary, sandalwood, sweet orange, yuzu

PRECAUTIONS

Avoid topical use during pregnancy due to increased risk of skin sensitization. Cypress essential oil gets stronger with age, so the older the oil, the less you'll need.

Frankincense

Boswellia carterii

SPICY, WOODY SCENT

COST: $$

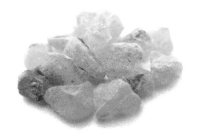

Frankincense has been used in incense for thousands of years, and it is also used as a remedy for a variety of skin ailments. Its ability to calm the mind and create inner peace makes it a valuable oil to diffuse during meditation, and its mildly sedative property encourages deep, slow breathing. Its expectorant and antiseptic properties make it ideal for helping with respiratory illnesses.

MEDICINAL PROPERTIES
Antiseptic, astringent, carminative, cicatrizant, cytophylactic, digestive, diuretic, emmenagogue, expectorant, sedative, vulnerary

USED FOR
Asthma, bronchitis, cough, cold, and laryngitis; ideal for making healing balms and salves for wounds, scars, aging skin, and inflammation

BLENDS WELL WITH
Bergamot, black pepper, cinnamon leaf, cypress, geranium, grapefruit, helichrysum, lavender, lemon, mandarin, neroli, orange, palmarosa, patchouli, pine, rose, rose geranium, sandalwood, vetiver, ylang-ylang

PRECAUTIONS
Do not use during pregnancy.

German Chamomile

Matricaria recutita

STRONG, SWEET,
  HERBACEOUS SCENT

COST: $$$

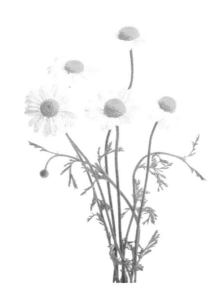

If you have ever spent time relaxing with a cup of hot chamomile tea, you have probably felt the wonderfully relaxing quality of German chamomile at work. Besides offering gentle sedation, particularly at bedtime or when suffering from a nasty cold, German chamomile contains levomenol, which helps heal compromised skin. Also known as blue chamomile, German chamomile essential oil gets its vivid color from azulene, which imparts a potent anti-inflammatory effect.

MEDICINAL PROPERTIES

Analgesic, antiallergenic, antibiotic, anti-inflammatory, antispasmodic, bactericidal, carminative, cholagogue, cicatrizant, digestive, emmenagogue, hepatic, sedative, stomachic, vasoconstrictor, vermifuge, vulnerary

USED FOR

Inflamed skin, psoriasis, and eczema

BLENDS WELL WITH

Benzoin, bergamot, clary sage, frankincense, geranium, grapefruit, helichrysum, jasmine, lavender, lemon, lime, mandarin, marjoram, neroli, patchouli, ravintsara, rose, rosemary, sweet orange, tea tree, ylang-ylang

PRECAUTIONS

Do not use during pregnancy.

Ginger

Zingiber officinale

WARM, SPICY SCENT

COST: $

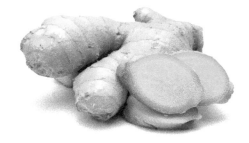

Ginger is a tropical perennial herb that bears fragrant flowers and a crown of narrow, spear-shaped leaves. Although it is prized for its aboveground beauty and aroma, the spice and essential oil come from its roots, which are thick, spreading rhizomes. Ginger has been used medicinally for millennia, with mentions in Chinese and Sanskrit texts as well as in ancient Roman, Greek, and Arabian literature. The plant's name is derived from India's Gingee district, where ginger tea is used to comfort upset stomachs.

MEDICINAL PROPERTIES
Analgesic, antiemetic, antiseptic, antispasmodic, bactericidal, carminative, cephalic, expectorant, febrifuge, laxative, rubefacient, stimulant, stomachic, sudorific

USED FOR
Nausea, vomiting, hangovers, and travel sickness; ideal for making pain-relieving salves for sore joints and muscles

BLENDS WELL WITH
Allspice, anise, Atlas cedarwood, bergamot, cedarwood, clove bud, coriander, eucalyptus (all species), frankincense, galbanum, geranium, grapefruit, jasmine, juniper berry, lemon, lime, mandarin, neroli, palmarosa, patchouli, rose, sweet orange, vetiver, ylang-ylang, yuzu

PRECAUTIONS
Not recommended for use during pregnancy due to increased risk of skin sensitization. Ginger can cause skin irritation and can be phototoxic; do not apply to skin that will be exposed to direct sunlight.

Helichrysum

Helichrysum italicum

STRONG, HERBAL SCENT

COST: $$$

Helichrysum essential oil isn't cheap, but it is a powerful addition to your aromatherapy arsenal. Sourced from an aromatic evergreen, it is also known as immortelle or everlasting. Traditional uses for this Mediterranean plant include applications for allergies, colds and coughs, wound healing, indigestion, and much more.

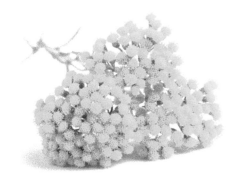

MEDICINAL PROPERTIES
Analgesic, anti-allergenic, anti-bacterial, antidepressant, antifungal, anti-inflammatory, antiseptic, anti-spasmodic, antitussive, antiviral, astringent, cholagogue, cytophylactic, diuretic, emollient, expectorant, hepatic, nervine, sedative, skin regenerator

USED FOR
Chronic skin conditions, bruises, acne, and arthritis; ideal for making first aid salves and stretch mark balms

BLENDS WELL WITH
Bergamot, black pepper, clary sage, clove bud, cypress, frankincense, galbanum, geranium, German chamomile, lavender, mandarin, oregano, Roman chamomile, rosewood, sweet orange, tea tree, vetiver, yuzu

PRECAUTIONS
Generally regarded as safe.

Lavender

Lavandula angustifolia

HERBACEOUS, FLORAL SCENT

COST: $

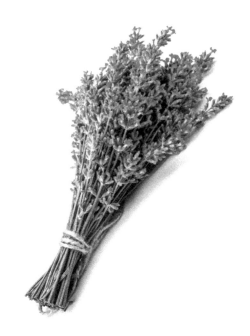

Lavender is among the most versatile of all essential oils, thanks to its ability to soothe pain, help wounds heal faster, and ease you into deep, relaxing sleep. Lavender gets its name from the Latin word *lavare*, meaning "to wash," and Romans used it extensively in bathing. It was the Romans who introduced lavender to England, where it remains a favorite today.

MEDICINAL PROPERTIES

Analgesic, antidepressant, anti-inflammatory, antiseptic, antispasmodic, antiviral, bactericide, carminative, cholagogue, cicatrizant, cordial, cytophylactic, decongestant, deodorant, diuretic, hypotensive, nervine, rubefacient, sedative, sudorific, vulnerary

USED FOR

Minor burns, cuts, and bruises; ideal for making soothing bedtime bath salts, lotions, and linen sprays

BLENDS WELL WITH

Atlas cedarwood, cedarwood, clary sage, cypress, galbanum, geranium, juniper berry, lemongrass, melissa, peppermint, pine, rosemary, spearmint, tagetes

PRECAUTIONS

Generally regarded as safe. Allergic reactions can develop with overuse; discontinue if irritation occurs.

Lemon

Citrus limonum

SHARP, CITRUS SCENT

COST: $

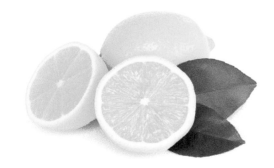

In Japan, lemon essential oil is often diffused in banks and other businesses where sharp attention to detail is required, because the crisp aroma helps promote alertness. Sourced from the same trees that provide the tangy, vitamin-rich citrus fruit that goes into popular beverages, candies, and culinary treats, lemon essential oil is a pleasant and useful addition to your aromatherapy kit.

MEDICINAL PROPERTIES

Antiseptic, bactericidal, carminative, cicatrizant, depurative, diaphoretic, diuretic, febrifuge, hemostatic, hypotensive, insecticidal, rubefacient, tonic, vermifuge

USED FOR

Bronchitis, asthma, and respiratory infections; ideal for making bath and body products as well as cleaning products

BLENDS WELL WITH

Allspice, benzoin, caraway seed, cardamom, eucalyptus (all types), fennel seed, geranium, juniper berry, neroli, Ravensara leaf, ravintsara, rose, rose geranium, rosewood, tagetes

PRECAUTIONS

Phototoxic; do not apply to skin that will be exposed to direct sunlight. Lemon can cause sensitive skin.

Lemongrass

Cymbopogon citratus,
C. flexuosus

GREEN, CITRUS SCENT

COST: $

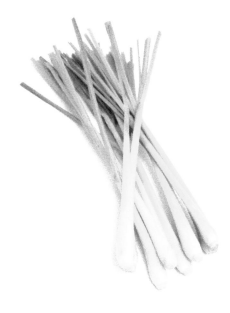

Lemongrass is a popular ingredient in Asian cuisine, and the essential oil often makes its way into natural insect repellents. This aromatic grass is a native of India, where it grows wild and reaches a height of about three feet. It is prized in Ayurvedic medicine for its ability to combat infections and reduce fevers.

MEDICINAL PROPERTIES
Analgesic, antidepressant, antimicrobial, antiseptic, astringent, bactericidal, carminative, deodorant, diuretic, febrifuge, fungicidal, galactagogue, insect repellent, insecticidal, nervine

USED FOR
Jet lag, headaches, and stress; ideal for making insect repellent and antifungal bath and body products

BLENDS WELL WITH
Basil, cajuput, coriander, geranium, jasmine, lavandin, lavender, palmarosa, patchouli, tea tree, vetiver

PRECAUTIONS
Do not use on children younger than two years old. Lemongrass can irritate diseased, damaged, or hypersensitive skin.

Myrtle

Myrtus communis

LIGHT, FRESH SCENT

COST: $$

Myrtle has long been a **representative of** peace, love, and **harmony**; in Britain, it often finds its way into **bridal bouquets.** Ancient Romans and **Greeks valued** it for its ability to relieve a **litany of** digestive complaints. Myrtle **essential** oil addresses a wide range of ail**ments**, yet it is mild enough for young **children** and seniors.

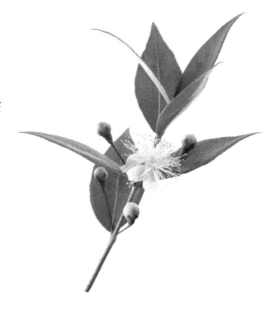

MEDICINAL PROPERTIES
Antibacterial, antifungal, anti-inflammatory, antimicrobial, antioxidant, antiseptic, antispasmodic, astringent, decongestant, deodorant, digestive, diuretic, emmenagogue, expectorant, laxative, nervine, sedative

BLENDS WELL WITH
Allspice, bay laurel, bergamot, cinnamon leaf, clary sage, clove bud, cypress, ginger, hyssop, lime, melissa, neroli, rosemary

USED FOR
Coughs, cold and flu symptoms, and abdominal issues; ideal for making skin care products to sort out acne, psoriasis, and irritation

PRECAUTIONS
Do not use during pregnancy.

Palmarosa

Cymbopogon martinii

SWEET, FLORAL SCENT

COST: $

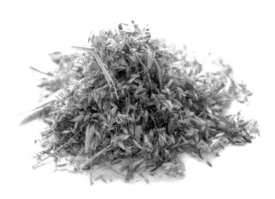

Although palmarosa is sometimes referred to as Turkish or East Indian geranium, it comes from a wild-growing grass with straw-colored leaves and flowering tops. Despite its floral scent, the herb is harvested before the flowers appear. Palmarosa is used commercially to scent tobacco, soaps, cosmetics, and perfumes.

MEDICINAL PROPERTIES

Analgesic, antiseptic, antiviral, bactericide, cicatrizant, cytophylactic, digestive, febrifuge

USED FOR

Digestive issues, and cold and flu; ideal for making nourishing skin care blends that address acne and dermatitis while regenerating skin

BLENDS WELL WITH

Bergamot, geranium, lemon, lime, mandarin, melissa, neroli, patchouli, petitgrain, Ravensara leaf, rose, rose geranium, rosemary, rosewood, sweet orange, tangerine, ylang-ylang, yuzu

PRECAUTIONS

Generally regarded as safe.

Patchouli

Pogostemon cablin

SWEET, SPICY, WOODY SCENT

COST: $$

Arguably one of the most intriguing of scents, patchouli became popular when textile companies began using it to repel lice and fleas in fabric used to make clothing and bedding. It was also used to give India ink its signature smell. Patchouli has a long history of masking unpleasant odors and serving as a base note in perfumes; despite its popularity in aromatic applications, it offers a wide range of medicinal properties.

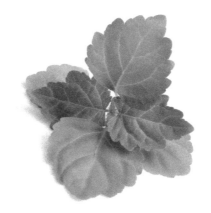

MEDICINAL PROPERTIES
Antidepressant, antiemetic, antifungal, anti-inflammatory, antimicrobial, antiseptic, antiviral, aphrodisiac, astringent, calmative, carminative, cicatrizant, deodorant, digestive, diuretic, febrifuge, fungicidal, insect repellent, insecticide, sedative

BLENDS WELL WITH
Bergamot, clary sage, davana, geranium, lavender, mandarin, myrrh, palmarosa, rose geranium, Spanish sage, spikenard, sweet orange, tangerine, yuzu

PRECAUTIONS
Generally regarded as safe.

USED FOR
Hemorrhoids, yeast infections, and fungal infections, including athlete's foot; ideal for use in perfumes and skin care products

Rose Geranium

Pelargonium graveolens

GREEN, FLORAL SCENT

COST: $$

Sometimes referred to as bourbon geranium, rose geranium has a light, rosy scent with minty undertones. Rose geranium's ability to stimulate the adrenal cortex (the outer part of the adrenal gland) makes it useful in lifting depression and alleviating anxiety. It stimulates the lymph system to aid in detoxification, and it helps balance dry and oily skin.

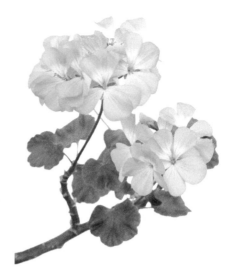

MEDICINAL PROPERTIES

Antidepressant, antiseptic, astringent, cicatrizant, cytophylactic, deodorant, diuretic, hemostatic, styptic, vermifuge, vulnerary

USED FOR

Sunburn, PMS, and painful periods; ideal for making nourishing bath and body products

BLENDS WELL WITH

Basil, bergamot, carrot seed, cedarwood, citronella, clary sage, cucumber seed, grapefruit, jasmine, lavender, lemon, lime, mandarin, neroli, patchouli, rosemary, sweet orange

PRECAUTIONS

Not recommended for use during pregnancy due to rose geranium's hormone-balancing properties.

Rosemary

Rosmarinus officinalis

REFRESHING, HERBAL SCENT

COST: $

Rosemary has the intriguing ability to stimulate memory and facilitate clear thinking. In ancient Greece, scholars wore rosemary while studying, as it helped them retain information. Diffusing rosemary essential oil can sharpen your focus, aid with productivity, and promote a sense of calm confidence.

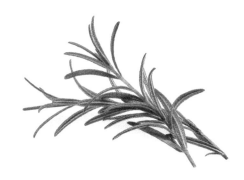

MEDICINAL PROPERTIES

Analgesic, antibacterial, antidepressant, antifungal, antimicrobial, antioxidant, antiseptic, antispasmodic, astringent, carminative, cicatrizant, digestive, diuretic, emmenagogue, hepatic, hypertensive, stimulant, sudorific, vulnerary

USED FOR

Digestive complaints, muscle pain, thinning hair, and dandruff; ideal for making bath and body products to balance skin and nourish hair

BLENDS WELL WITH

Balsam of Peru, basil, bay laurel, bergamot, cajuput, clary sage, clove bud, elemi, fennel seed, juniper berry, lemon, niaouli, peppermint, petitgrain, Spanish sage, spearmint, tea tree

PRECAUTIONS

Do not use during pregnancy. Do not use if diagnosed with epilepsy. Rosemary is quite stimulating; using it within three to four hours of bedtime can cause wakefulness.

Spearmint

Mentha spicata, M. viridis

SWEET, MINTY SCENT

COST: $

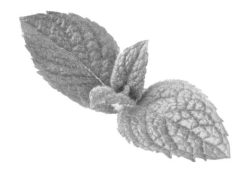

A gentler substitute for peppermint essential oil, spearmint calms itching, relieves coughs and colds, eases indigestion, and has a marvelously uplifting effect on the mind. A Mediterranean native that is now cultivated worldwide, spearmint was used by ancient Greeks, who enjoyed the scent in their bathwater. During medieval times, it was used to whiten teeth and soothe sore gums, much in the way we use fresh, minty toothpaste today.

MEDICINAL PROPERTIES

Antidepressant, antiseptic, antispasmodic, astringent, carminative, cephalic, decongestant, digestive, diuretic, expectorant, insecticide, stimulant, stomachic

USED FOR

Halitosis, hiccups, and headaches; ideal for making balms to fight acne and relieve itching

BLENDS WELL WITH

Basil, bay laurel, benzoin, eucalyptus (any species), jasmine, lavender, lemon, lime, mandarin, niaouli, peppermint, rosemary, sweet orange, tangerine

PRECAUTIONS

Do not use spearmint if breastfeeding, as it can reduce lactation. Spearmint is unique in that it can sometimes weaken homeopathic remedies; if you take a homeopathic remedy, ensure that spearmint is compatible before using it.

Sweet Basil

Ocimum basilicum

SWEET, HERBACEOUS SCENT

COST: $

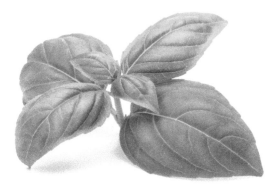

Sweet basil essential oil comes from the common culinary herb, which gets its name from the Greek word *basileum*, meaning king. It is a fantastic skin tonic, and it can lessen the pain of menstrual cramps, rheumatism, gout, and sore muscles. Sweet basil should be avoided during pregnancy. However, when nursing, its use promotes milk production. In Italy, new moms traditionally eat basil leaves to stimulate lactation.

MEDICINAL PROPERTIES

Antibacterial, antidepressant, antiseptic, antispasmodic, digestive, expectorant, restorative, stomachic

USED FOR

Migraines, eliminating anxiousness, and soothing insect bites

BLENDS WELL WITH

Bay laurel, black pepper, citronella, lemon, lemongrass, lime, marjoram, melissa, oregano, peppermint, ravintsara, spearmint, vetiver, yuzu

PRECAUTIONS

Do not use during pregnancy.

Sweet Marjoram

Origanum majorana

SWEET, SPICY SCENT

COST: $

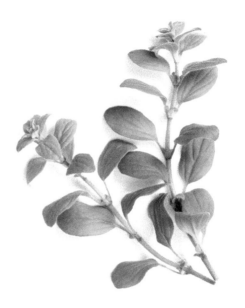

Also known as knotted marjoram, *Origanum majorana* originated in North Africa and the Mediterranean and reached Egypt sometime around 2000 BCE. The herb was dedicated to Osiris, the Egyptian god of the underworld, and it was used in funerary preparations as well as in love potions and medicines. Sweet marjoram is a very relaxing essential oil, and it's a good choice for soothing the symptoms of cold, flu, and digestive ailments.

MEDICINAL PROPERTIES

Analgesic, antiseptic, antispasmodic, antiviral, bactericidal, carminative, cephalic, cordial, diaphoretic, digestive, diuretic, emmenagogue, expectorant, fungicidal, hypotensive, laxative, nervine, sedative, stomachic, vasodilator, vulnerary

USED FOR

Effective in lessening the symptoms of congestion and sinusitis; ideal for use in warming blends to ease muscle pain

BLENDS WELL WITH

Atlas cedarwood, bergamot, black pepper, cedarwood, clary sage, cypress, German chamomile, lavender, lemon, lime, myrtle, ravensara leaf, Roman chamomile, rosemary, sweet orange

PRECAUTIONS

Do not use during pregnancy.

Sweet Orange

Citrus sinensis

SWEET, CITRUS SCENT

COST: $

Oranges make a fantastic snack, but historically, they have also been put to medicinal and cosmetic uses. In ancient China, dried oranges were a popular remedy for a bloated stomach, and the peel was used to relieve coughing. Sweet orange's enticing aroma is good for more than just air fresheners; it (and that of other citrus oils) have been successfully used to curb cigarette cravings.

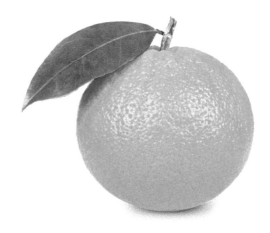

MEDICINAL PROPERTIES

Antibacterial, antidepressant, anti-inflammatory, antiseptic, antiviral, aperitif, astringent, carminative, cholagogue, digestive, diuretic, fungicidal, hypotensive, stomachic, tonic

USED FOR

Cold, flu, and digestive ailments; ideal for making air fresheners and cleaning products

BLENDS WELL WITH

Anise, allspice, black pepper, caraway seed, cardamom, cinnamon leaf, clove bud, copaiba, elemi, fennel seed, frankincense, galbanum, ginger, rosewood, sandalwood, tagetes, vetiver

PRECAUTIONS

Phototoxic; do not apply to skin that will be exposed to direct sunlight. Use it within six months of opening for topical use, and reserve older oil for inhalation and household cleaning purposes.

Tea Tree

Melaleuca alternifolia

LIGHT, CAMPHOR SCENT

COST: $

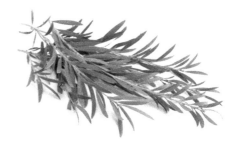

One of the most potent immune-stimulating essential oils available, tea tree comes from New South Wales in Australia, where aboriginal people first enjoyed its many medicinal purposes. During World War II, tea tree was so important to the Allies that tea tree cutters and producers were exempt from military service. Soldiers and sailors used it the same way as it is employed today—to help heal minor wounds, infections, and more.

MEDICINAL PROPERTIES

Antimicrobial, antiseptic, antiviral, bactericide, cicatrizant, expectorant, fungicide, insect repellent, insecticide, stimulant, sudorific

USED FOR

Minor wounds, sinusitis, and respiratory ailments; ideal for making powerful anti-septic household cleaners

BLENDS WELL WITH

Cinnamon leaf, clary sage, clove bud, eucalyptus (any species), geranium, lavender, lemon, myrrh, oregano, rosemary, rosewood, thyme

PRECAUTIONS

Generally regarded as safe.

Thyme

Thymus vulgaris

SPICY, HERBACEOUS SCENT

COST: $$

Thyme has a long history of culinary use as well as an interesting medicinal background. Ancient Greeks used it to repel insects, and Romans believed bathing in thyme-scented water would impart courage and vigor. Thyme is a spicy oil that must be used judiciously. In salves and compresses, it increases circulation, making it ideal for helping with sprains, bruises, and muscle aches.

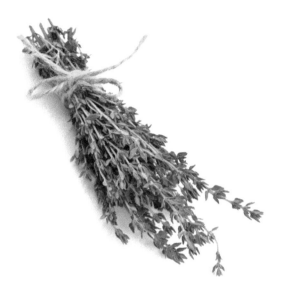

MEDICINAL PROPERTIES

Antibacterial, antifungal, antimicrobial, antioxidant, antiseptic, antispasmodic, antitoxic, antitussive, astringent, cicatrizant, disinfectant, expectorant, hypertensive, insect repellent, insecticide, stimulant, sudorific

USED FOR

Diarrhea, infectious colitis, and upper respiratory infections; ideal for making insect repellents

BLENDS WELL WITH

Balsam of Peru, bay laurel, bergamot, black pepper, clary sage, fir needle, grapefruit, juniper berry, lemon, lime, lavender, pine, rosemary, Spanish sage

PRECAUTIONS

Do not use on children younger than six years old.

Vetiver

Chrysopogon zizanioides

SWEET, WOODY SCENT

COST: $

Vetiver is a tufted perennial grass native to the tropics, where it is used to weave fragrant mats, baskets, and window coverings and also for erosion control in wet areas. Besides its many practical uses, vetiver is widely employed by the fragrance industry. In aromatherapy, it is called the "oil of tranquility" for its ability to ward off depression and calm nervousness and stress.

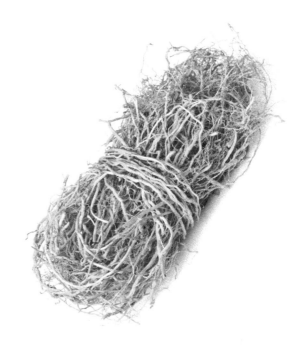

MEDICINAL PROPERTIES

Analgesic, anti-inflammatory, antiseptic, antispasmodic, aphrodisiac, astringent, calmative, cicatrizant, detoxifier, insect repellent, nervine, sedative, stomachic, tonic, vulnerary

BLENDS WELL WITH

Benzoin, cardamom, clary sage, fennel seed, grapefruit, jasmine, mandarin, marjoram, may chang, neroli, patchouli, petitgrain, sweet orange, tangerine, ylang-ylang

USED FOR

Attention deficit hyperactivity disorder, stress, and postpartum depression; ideal for making soothing products to ease the pain of arthritis, rheumatism, muscle strains, and more

PRECAUTIONS

Generally regarded as safe.

White Pine

Pinus strobus

FRESH, GREEN-FOREST SCENT

COST: $

Native Americans and others have used white pine's rich, delicious seeds as a source of protein and fat and have employed its needles as a source of vitamin C. It can lessen arthritis, muscle, and joint pain, and in those with respiratory illnesses it can help focus breathing.

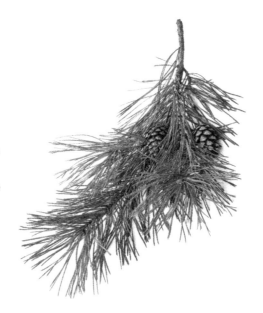

MEDICINAL PROPERTIES

Analgesic, antibacterial, antiseptic, antiviral, cholagogue, deodorant, diuretic, expectorant, insecticide, rubefacient, stimulant, sudorific, vermifuge

USED FOR

Effective in treating cold, cough, sinusitis, and bronchitis; ideal for making soothing salves to ease muscle and joint pain

BLENDS WELL WITH

Atlas cedarwood, bay laurel, cedarwood, clary sage, eucalyptus (all species), fir needle, juniper, lavender, lemon, niaouli, ravensara leaf, rosemary, Spanish sage, spikenard

PRECAUTIONS

Not recommended for use during pregnancy due to the increased risk of skin sensitization. White pine can cause skin irritation.

Yarrow

Achillea millefolium

SWEET, PENETRATING,
   HERBACEOUS SCENT

COST: $

Also known as milfoil, common yarrow, and thousand leaf, this oil is extracted from *Achillea millefolium* and is a member of the *Asteraceae* plant family. Yarrow can grow up to three feet tall and is a perennial herb known throughout North America, Europe, and Asia. Yarrow produces aromatic, feathery leaves with pink and white flowers.

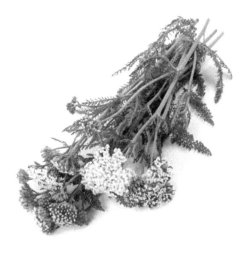

MEDICINAL PROPERTIES
Anti-inflammatory, astringent, antispasmodic, digestive, expectorant, hypotensive

USED FOR
Poor circulation, inflammation, toxins, and arthritis

BLENDS WELL WITH
Chamomile, peppermint, frankincense, helichrysum

PRECAUTIONS
Do not use if pregnant, breastfeeding, or epileptic. Do not use with young children. Do not take orally.

Ylang-ylang

Cananga odorata

SWEET FLORAL SCENT

COST: $$

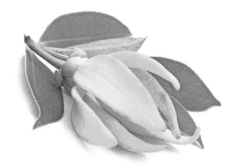

Sometimes referred to as "poor man's jasmine," ylang-ylang has a beautifully haunting scent that makes it a favorite with perfumeries. Pronounced "ee-lang ee-lang," *ylang-ylang* means "flower of flowers." Like jasmine, neroli, and other heady florals, a little bit goes a long way.

MEDICINAL PROPERTIES

Antidepressant, antiseborrheic, antiseptic, aphrodisiac, hypotensive, nervine, sedative

USED FOR

Stress, nervousness, and anxiety; ideal for making romantic and relaxing bath and body products

BLENDS WELL WITH

Bergamot, cypress, davana, grapefruit, lavender, lemon, mandarin, petitgrain, rosewood, sandalwood, tangerine, vetiver, yuzu

PRECAUTIONS

Generally regarded as safe; however, overuse can cause nausea and headaches.

Essential Oils Labor Kit

Whether it's a home birth or a hospital birth, every woman needs a basic essential oils labor kit to tackle whatever comes her way.

CLARY SAGE Though it is contraindicated during pregnancy, clary sage essential oil is a must-have during labor. It encourages and strengthens contractions, relieves muscular pain, and eases stress and anxiety.

GRAPEFRUIT This refreshing and uplifting essential oil is not only antibacterial and antiseptic, but also raises spirits while calming nervous fears and anxiety. Grapefruit essential oil can help with nausea and vomiting during labor as well.

LAVENDER This multifaceted essential oil can be used during nearly every stage of labor to ease pain and calm nervous fears. Lavender essential oil is naturally antiseptic and antibacterial and can be used to kill germs on hands and in the air.

ROMAN CHAMOMILE Calming and soothing, chamomile essential oil is not just an anti-inflammatory, but also a natural digestive and can help with nausea during labor. This happy essential oil mixes well with grapefruit essential oil and can help lift the mood in the room when things get tense.

ROSALINA Gentle and multifaceted like lavender, this cleansing essential oil is naturally antibacterial and antiseptic. Used as a gentle substitute for eucalyptus, when diffused, rosalina cleanses the air and can support healthy breathing. Also used as a natural pain reliever, diluting rosalina in a carrier oil and massaging onto the belly and back helps ease some of the labor pain.

SPEARMINT The gentler version of peppermint, spearmint is great to keep on hand for any nausea or vomiting during labor. When diffused, this uplifting, happy essential oil reduces stress and anxiety while improving focus.

Ailments and Oils
Quick-Reference Guide

PREGNANCY

AILMENT	SUGGESTED ESSENTIAL OILS	METHODS OF APPLICATION
Acne	Cedarwood, chamomile, geranium, lavender, palmarosa, rosalina, sweet orange, tea tree	STEAM, TOPICAL
Allergies (Hay Fever)	Blue tansy, chamomile (German), cypress, fir needle, frankincense, lavender, lemon, rosalina, sweet orange	INHALATION, STEAM
Anxiety	Bergamot, cedarwood, chamomile, coriander, grapefruit, lavender, lemon, neroli, sandalwood, sweet orange, vanilla, ylang-ylang	INHALATION, ROOM SPRAY, TOPICAL
Backaches	Black pepper, cypress, fir needle, helichrysum, juniper, lavender, marjoram, rosalina, spearmint	BATH, TOPICAL
Breast Tenderness	Chamomile, cypress, frankincense, geranium, grapefruit, helichrysum, lavender, marjoram, rosalina, ylang-ylang	MASSAGE, TOPICAL
Carpal Tunnel Syndrome	Cypress, frankincense, ginger, helichrysum, lavender, marjoram, rosalina, spearmint, turmeric CO_2	MASSAGE, TOPICAL
Cold and Flu	Blue tansy, chamomile, citrus, cypress, fir needle, frankincense, juniper, lavender, marjoram, palmarosa, pine, rosalina, spearmint, spruce, tea tree	BATH, COMPRESS, INHALATION
Constipation	Chamomile, dill weed, frankincense, ginger, lemon, petitgrain, spearmint, sweet orange	MASSAGE, TOPICAL

AILMENT	SUGGESTED ESSENTIAL OILS	METHODS OF APPLICATION
Cough	Blue tansy, chamomile, cypress, fir needle, frankincense, lavender, lemon, pine, rosalina, spearmint, spruce, tea tree	INHALATION, TOPICAL
Depression	Bergamot, chamomile, clary sage, frankincense, geranium, grapefruit, lavender, neroli, patchouli, petitgrain, sandalwood, sweet orange, ylang-ylang	INHALATION
Dizziness	Chamomile, cypress, fir needle, frankincense, ginger, grapefruit, juniper, lavender, lemon, rosalina, spearmint, sweet orange	INHALATION
Ear Infection	Chamomile, frankincense, lavender, marjoram, palmarosa, rosalina, tea tree	TOPICAL
Edema and Swelling	Chamomile, cypress, geranium, ginger, grapefruit, juniper, lavender, lemon, rosalina, spearmint, tea tree	BATH, MASSAGE, TOPICAL
Fetal Positioning	Rosalina, spearmint	MASSAGE, TOPICAL
Group B Strep/ Bacterial Vaginosis	Lavender, palmarosa, rosalina, tea tree	BATH, TOPICAL
Headaches	Black pepper, blue tansy, chamomile, cypress, fir needle, frankincense, helichrysum, juniper, lavender, marjoram, neroli, petitgrain, rosalina, spearmint	BATH, INHALATION, MASSAGE, TOPICAL
Heartburn	Bergamot, chamomile, coriander, cypress, ginger, grapefruit, lavender, lemon, marjoram, neroli, sweet orange, spearmint	INHALATION, TOPICAL
Hemorrhoids	Cedarwood, chamomile, cypress, frankincense, geranium, helichrysum, juniper, sandalwood	BATH, TOPICAL

AILMENT	SUGGESTED ESSENTIAL OILS	METHODS OF APPLICATION
Insomnia	Bergamot, cedarwood, chamomile, coriander, frankincense, lavender, mandarin, petitgrain, sandalwood, sweet orange, vetiver	BATH, INHALATION, MASSAGE, TOPICAL
Leg Cramps	Chamomile, cypress, fir needle, frankincense, helichrysum, juniper, lavender, lemon, marjoram, petitgrain, rosalina	BATH, MASSAGE, TOPICAL
Morning Sickness	Bergamot, chamomile, ginger, grapefruit, lemon, petitgrain, spearmint, sweet orange	INHALATION
Preeclampsia	Bergamot, blue tansy, chamomile, coriander, frankincense, geranium, lavender, mandarin, petitgrain, rosalina, sandalwood, sweet orange, vetiver, ylang-ylang	INHALATION, MASSAGE, ROOM SPRAY, TOPICAL
Pregnancy Fatigue	Bergamot, coriander, cypress, fir needle, geranium, ginger, grapefruit, lemon, lemon eucalyptus, pine	INHALATION, MASSAGE, TOPICAL
PUPPP	Blue tansy, chamomile, geranium, helichrysum, lavender, patchouli, rosalina, sandalwood, spearmint	BATH, TOPICAL
Round Ligament Pains	Black pepper, blue tansy, chamomile, cypress, fir needle, frankincense, ginger, helichrysum, lavender, marjoram, petitgrain, rosalina, sandalwood, spearmint, ylang-ylang	MASSAGE, TOPICAL
Sciatica	Black pepper, cypress, fir needle, lavender, marjoram, petitgrain, rosalina, spearmint, turmeric	BATH, MASSAGE, TOPICAL
Stretch Marks	Blue tansy, chamomile, frankincense, geranium, helichrysum, lavender, lemon, neroli, patchouli, sandalwood	MASSAGE, TOPICAL

AILMENT	SUGGESTED ESSENTIAL OILS	METHODS OF APPLICATION
Urinary Tract Infections	Lavender, rosalina, tea tree	BATH, TOPICAL
Varicose Veins	Blue tansy, cedarwood, chamomile, cypress, fir needle, frankincense, geranium, ginger, grapefruit, helichrysum, juniper, lavender, lemon, neroli, rosalina, sandalwood	BATH, MASSAGE, TOPICAL
Yeast Infections	Cedarwood, chamomile, coriander, frankincense, geranium, grapefruit, lavender, lemon, mandarin, sweet orange, tangerine, tea tree	TOPICAL

LABOR AND DELIVERY, POSTPARTUM, AND BREASTFEEDING

AILMENT	SUGGESTED ESSENTIAL OILS	METHODS OF APPLICATION
After Pains	Balsam fir, bergamot, black pepper, chamomile, coriander, cypress, fir needle, geranium, ginger, helichrysum, jasmine, lavender, lemon, marjoram, petitgrain, rosalina, spruce, tangerine	COMPRESS, MASSAGE, TOPICAL
Anxiety	Bergamot, chamomile, clary sage, coriander, grapefruit, lavender, lemon, neroli, petitgrain, sandalwood, sweet orange, vanilla, ylang-ylang	INHALATION, ROOM SPRAY
Back Labor	Bergamot, black pepper, chamomile, coriander, cypress, fir needle, frankincense, ginger, helichrysum, lavender, lemon, marjoram, petitgrain, rosalina, tangerine, spruce	LINIMENT, MASSAGE, TOPICAL
Back Pains	Balsam fir, bergamot, black pepper, chamomile, coriander, cypress, fir needle, frankincense, ginger, helichrysum, lavender, lemon, marjoram, petitgrain, rosalina, tangerine, spruce, turmeric	LINIMENT, MASSAGE, TOPICAL

AILMENT	SUGGESTED ESSENTIAL OILS	METHODS OF APPLICATION
Blocked Ducts and Mastitis	Balsam fir, bergamot, black pepper, chamomile, coriander, cypress, fir needle, frankincense, ginger, helichrysum, lemon, lavender, marjoram, neroli, rosalina, spruce, tangerine	COMPRESS, MASSAGE, TOPICAL
Blood Pressure	Bergamot, blue tansy, cedarwood, chamomile, clary sage, coriander, frankincense, lavender, mandarin, marjoram, petitgrain, rosalina, sandalwood, tangerine, vanilla, vetiver, ylang-ylang	INHALATION
Contractions	Bergamot, chamomile, cedarwood, coriander, cypress, fir needle, frankincense, grapefruit, juniper, lavender, lemon, lemon eucalyptus, patchouli, petitgrain, rosalina, spearmint, sweet orange	INHALATION, MASSAGE, TOPICAL
C-Section Care	Cedarwood, chamomile, frankincense, geranium, helichrysum, lavender, lemon, neroli, palmarosa, sweet orange, tangerine	INHALATION, TOPICAL, WASH
Episiotomy Care	Chamomile, cypress, fir needle, frankincense, geranium, helichrysum, lavender, lemon, marjoram, palmarosa, patchouli, sandalwood, sweet orange, tangerine, tea tree	BATH, TOPICAL, WASH
Fatigue During Labor	Bergamot, black pepper, cedarwood, coriander, fir needle, geranium, ginger, grapefruit, juniper, lemon, palmarosa, petitgrain, pine, spearmint, spruce, sweet orange, tangerine	INHALATION, ROOM SPRAY
Germ Killing	Bergamot, cedarwood, chamomile, coriander, cypress, fir needle, frankincense, geranium, grapefruit, helichrysum, lavender, lemon, mandarin, marjoram, neroli, petitgrain, rosalina, sandalwood, sweet orange, tangerine	HAND SOAP, INHALATION, TOPICAL

AILMENT	SUGGESTED ESSENTIAL OILS	METHODS OF APPLICATION
Hair Loss	Black pepper, cedarwood, chamomile, clary sage, coriander, cypress, fir needle, frankincense, geranium, juniper, lavender, lemon, palmarosa, patchouli, pine, sandalwood, spearmint, sweet orange, tea tree, vetiver, ylang-ylang	MASSAGE, SPRAY, TOPICAL
Milk Production	Clary sage, fenugreek, geranium	LINIMENT, MASSAGE, TOPICAL
Nausea	Bergamot, chamomile, dill weed, ginger, grapefruit, lemon, mandarin, spearmint, sweet orange, tangerine	INHALATION, TOPICAL
Nipples (Dry/Cracked)	Blue tansy, chamomile, geranium, helichrysum, lavender, neroli, rose, sweet orange	TOPICAL
Postpartum Depression	Bergamot, cedarwood, chamomile, clary sage, coriander, geranium, grapefruit, lavender, lemon, neroli, petitgrain, sandalwood, sweet orange, vanilla, ylang-ylang	BODY SPRAY, INHALATION, TOPICAL
Postpartum Vaginal Care	Cedarwood, chamomile, cypress, fir needle, frankincense, helichrysum, lavender, lemon, mandarin, marjoram, neroli, patchouli, sandalwood, sweet orange, tea tree	BATH, COMPRESS, TOPICAL
Sore Breasts	Blue tansy, chamomile, frankincense, geranium, ginger, helichrysum, lavender, marjoram, patchouli, petitgrain, rosalina, sandalwood, ylang-ylang	COMPRESS, MASSAGE, TOPICAL
Speed Up Labor	Coriander, cypress, fir needle, frankincense, geranium, jasmine, juniper, lavender, rose, ylang-ylang	INHALATION
Transition	Bergamot, chamomile, clary sage, coriander, frankincense, lemon, mandarin, sweet orange, tangerine, vanilla	INHALATION, ROOM SPRAY, TOPICAL

INFANTS AND YOUNG CHILDREN

AILMENT	SUGGESTED ESSENTIAL OILS	METHODS OF APPLICATION
Allergies (Hay Fever)	Blue tansy, chamomile, citronella, cypress, fir needle, frankincense, grapefruit, juniper, lavender, lemon, pine, rosalina, spearmint, spruce, sweet orange	INHALATION
Anxiety	Bergamot, cedarwood, chamomile, coriander, frankincense, sandalwood, sweet orange, vanilla	INHALATION, MASSAGE, ROOM SPRAY, TOPICAL
Asthma	Blue tansy, chamomile, citronella, cypress, fir needle, frankincense, grapefruit, juniper, lavender, lemon, lemon eucalyptus, pine, rosalina, spearmint, spruce, sweet orange	BATH, INHALATION, TOPICAL
Athlete's Foot	Cedarwood, chamomile, coriander, frankincense, geranium, grapefruit, lavender, lemon, mandarin, pine, tangerine, tea tree	BATH, TOPICAL
Balanitis	Chamomile, geranium, lavender, palmarosa, tea tree	BATH, TOPICAL
Bedtime Fears	Chamomile, lavender, tangerine, vanilla	INHALATION, ROOM SPRAY
Blisters	Cedarwood, chamomile, cypress, fir needle, geranium, lavender, lemon, marjoram, neroli, palmarosa, petitgrain, rosalina, lavender, sweet orange, tea tree	BATH, TOPICAL, WASH
Bronchitis	Chamomile, cypress, fir needle, frankincense, ginger, lavender, lemon, marjoram, palmarosa, petitgrain, pine, rosalina, sandalwood, spearmint, spruce, tea tree	INHALATION, MASSAGE, SHOWER STEAMERS, TOPICAL
Bug Bites and Stings	Blue tansy, chamomile, coriander, cypress, frankincense, geranium, juniper, lavender, marjoram, neroli, palmarosa, patchouli, petitgrain, pine, rosalina, rose, sandalwood, spearmint, tea tree	TOPICAL

AILMENT	SUGGESTED ESSENTIAL OILS	METHODS OF APPLICATION
Bug Repellents	Cedarwood, geranium, grapefruit, lavender, lemon, mandarin, marjoram, patchouli, pine, rosalina, spearmint, sweet orange, tangerine, tea tree	BODY SPRAY, CANDLES, TOPICAL
Burns and Sunburns	Blue tansy, chamomile, frankincense, geranium, lavender, rosalina, spearmint	TOPICAL
Catarrh	Chamomile, cypress, fir needle, frankincense, ginger, lavender, marjoram, palmarosa, petitgrain, pine, rosalina, sandalwood, spearmint, spruce, tea tree	INHALATION, SALT STEAM, TOPICAL
Chicken pox	Coriander, frankincense, geranium, lavender, marjoram, neroli, palmarosa, petitgrain, rose, spearmint, sweet orange, tea tree	BATH, INHALATION, TOPICAL
Circumcision	Lavender hydrosol	COMPRESS, TOPICAL, WASH
Colds	Cinnamon, cypress, fir needle, frankincense, lavender, lemon, marjoram, palmarosa, rosalina, spearmint, tea tree	BATH, INHALATION, TOPICAL
Cold Sores	Chamomile, coriander, geranium, lavender, lemon, rosalina, tea tree	TOPICAL
Colic	Roman chamomile hydrosol	BATH, SPRAY, TOPICAL
Congestion	Cedarwood, cypress, fir needle, frankincense, juniper, lavender, lemon, lemon eucalyptus, rosalina, pine, spearmint, spruce, tea tree	INHALATION, SALT STEAM
Constipation	Chamomile, coriander, dill weed, frankincense, ginger, lemon, petitgrain, spearmint, sweet orange	MASSAGE, TOPICAL

AILMENT	SUGGESTED ESSENTIAL OILS	METHODS OF APPLICATION
Cough	Chamomile, cypress, fir needle, frankincense, ginger, lavender, marjoram, petitgrain, pine, rosalina, sandalwood, spearmint, spruce	INHALATION, MASSAGE, TOPICAL
Cradle Cap	Lavender hydrosol	TOPICAL
Croup	Black pepper, cedarwood, chamomile, cypress, frankincense, lavender, lemon, marjoram, palmarosa, pine, rosalina, sandalwood, spruce	INHALATION, MASSAGE, TOPICAL
Cuts and Scrapes	Blue tansy, cedarwood, chamomile, cypress, fir needle, frankincense, geranium, helichrysum, lavender, lemon, palmarosa, rose, sweet orange, tea tree	TOPICAL, WASH
Dandruff	Bergamot, cedarwood, chamomile, cinnamon, coriander, fir needle, geranium, grapefruit, lavender, lemon, palmarosa, patchouli, petitgrain, rosalina, sandalwood, sweet orange, tangerine, tea tree	SPRAY, TOPICAL
Diaper Rash	Blue tansy, chamomile, frankincense, geranium, lavender, lemon, neroli, palmarosa, petitgrain, rosalina, sweet orange	TOPICAL, WASH
Diarrhea	Chamomile, dill weed, ginger, lavender, lemon, petitgrain, spearmint, sweet orange	MASSAGE, TOPICAL
Dry Skin	Blue tansy, carrot seed, cedarwood, chamomile, coriander, frankincense, geranium, grapefruit, helichrysum, lavender, lemon, palmarosa, patchouli, petitgrain, rosalina, rose, sandalwood, sweet orange	TOPICAL
Earaches and Ear Infections	Chamomile, frankincense, lavender, marjoram, palmarosa, rosalina, tea tree	MASSAGE, TOPICAL

AILMENT	SUGGESTED ESSENTIAL OILS	METHODS OF APPLICATION
Eczema and Psoriasis	Blue tansy, cedarwood, chamomile, coriander, frankincense, geranium, helichrysum, lavender, neroli, palmarosa, patchouli, tea tree	TOPICAL, WASH
Fever	Chamomile, coriander, cypress, fir needle, grapefruit, lavender, lemon, marjoram, neroli, palmarosa, petitgrain, rosalina, spearmint, tea tree	BATH, COMPRESS
Germ Killing and Immune Boosting	Bergamot, cedarwood, chamomile, coriander, cypress, frankincense, geranium, grapefruit, helichrysum, lavender, lemon, mandarin, marjoram, neroli, petitgrain, rosalina, sandalwood, sweet orange, tangerine, tea tree	INHALATION, TOPICAL
Growing Pains	Chamomile, coriander, cypress, fir needle, helichrysum, juniper, lavender, lemon, marjoram, rosalina, turmeric	BATH, MASSAGE, TOPICAL
Hand, Foot, and Mouth Disease	Chamomile, coriander, geranium, helichrysum, lavender, neroli, palmarosa, petitgrain, rosalina, sandalwood, sweet orange, tea tree	TOPICAL, WASH
Headaches	Black pepper, blue tansy, chamomile, cypress, fir needle, frankincense, ginger, helichrysum, juniper, lavender, marjoram, neroli, petitgrain, rosalina, spearmint	INHALATION, TOPICAL
Head Lice	Cedarwood, geranium, lavender, palmarosa, patchouli, rosalina, spearmint, sweet orange, tea tree	TOPICAL
Heat Rash and Heat Exhaustion	Bergamot, blue tansy, chamomile, clary sage, cypress, fir needle, juniper, lemon, palmarosa, rosalina, spearmint	BATH, COMPRESS, SPRAY
Hives	Blue tansy, chamomile, helichrysum, lavender, lemon, neroli, palmarosa, rosalina, tea tree	COMPRESS, TOPICAL

AILMENT	SUGGESTED ESSENTIAL OILS	METHODS OF APPLICATION
Influenza	Bergamot, blue tansy, chamomile, cinnamon leaf, coriander, cypress, fir needle, grapefruit, juniper, lavender, lemon, marjoram, palmarosa, petitgrain, rosalina, sweet orange, tangerine, tea tree	INHALATION, TOPICAL
Nausea and Vomiting	Bergamot, chamomile, dill weed, ginger, grapefruit, lemon, mandarin, spearmint, sweet orange, tangerine	INHALATION
Pneumonia	Cedarwood, coriander, chamomile, cypress, fir needle, frankincense, ginger, juniper, lavender, lemon, lemon eucalyptus, marjoram, palmarosa, petitgrain, rosalina, spearmint, sweet orange, tea tree	INHALATION, SHOWER STEAMERS, TOPICAL
Poison Ivy, Oak, and Sumac	Blue tansy, chamomile, cypress, fir needle, frankincense, geranium, juniper, neroli, pine, lavender, marjoram, neroli, palmarosa, patchouli, rosalina, rose, sandalwood, spearmint, tea tree	BATH, TOPICAL
Ringworm	Cedarwood, chamomile, coriander, frankincense, geranium, grapefruit, lavender, mandarin, rosalina, sweet orange, tangerine, tea tree	TOPICAL
Sleep	Bergamot, cedarwood, chamomile, clary sage, coriander, frankincense, lavender, lemon, mandarin, marjoram, neroli, petitgrain, rosalina, sandalwood, sweet orange, tangerine, valerian root, vanilla, ylang-ylang	BATH, INHALATION, MASSAGE, TOPICAL
Sneezing	Blue tansy, chamomile, cypress, fir needle, geranium, juniper, lavender, lemon, rosalina, rose, spearmint	INHALATION
Sniffles and Runny Nose	Blue tansy, cedarwood, chamomile, cypress, fir needle, juniper, lavender, lemon, marjoram, palmarosa, rosalina, spearmint, spruce, tea tree	INHALATION

AILMENT	SUGGESTED ESSENTIAL OILS	METHODS OF APPLICATION
Sore Throat	Chamomile, frankincense, geranium, ginger, helichrysum, lavender, lemon, marjoram, rosalina, spearmint, tea tree	SPRAY, TOPICAL
Teething	Chamomile, lavender	TOPICAL
Thrush	Blue tansy, chamomile, frankincense, geranium, helichrysum, lavender, lemon, neroli, palmarosa, petitgrain, rosalina, spearmint, sweet orange, tea tree	TOPICAL
Umbilical Cord Infections	Lavender hydrosol	TOPICAL
Warts	Cedarwood, cypress, geranium, lavender, lemon, marjoram, rosalina, tea tree	TOPICAL

Known Prescription Interactions

There have been several case reports regarding extensive topical use of preparations containing high levels of the essential oil component methyl salicylate enhancing the effects of the anticoagulants warfarin and heparin, which led to extensive bleeding and hemorrhaging. Methyl salicylate is found in significant quantities in wintergreen and sweet birch essential oils, both of which have been listed as "potentially hazardous" in this book and whose use has been advised against. Therefore, further caution is advised with the topical use of essential oils high in methyl salicylate, such as wintergreen or sweet birch, especially if you are currently taking anticoagulants.

In addition, many common components of essential oils have demonstrated the capacity to enhance drug absorption via the skin, which could lead to toxic outcomes. If you are on prescribed medications that are delivered via skin patches, essential oil safety experts recommend to not use essential oils on the skin near, adjacent to, or under where conventional drug patches are being placed.

Although essential oils used topically or aromatically are unlikely to interfere with pharmaceuticals, internal and oral use of essential oils can pose a more significant interaction risk. The internal and oral use of essential oils has not been explored or recommended in this book, and the heightened risk of drug interactions emphasizes the need to work with a qualified health professional if you are considering using essential oils for internal use.

If you are ill and are currently taking pharmaceutical medications, it is advised that you speak to your doctor or other qualified health professional prior to integrating essential oils into your life.

References

Ablard, Kelly M. "Conservation of Essential Oil-, Carrier Oil-, and Extract-Bearing Plants." Accessed March 28, 2019. https://www.kellyablard.com/conservation /conservation-of-essential-oil-and-carrier-oil-bearing-plants/.

AromaWeb. "Hazardous Essential Oils." Accessed April 4, 2019. https://www .aromaweb.com/essentialoils/hazardous.asp.

Arslan, Dilek Efe, Sevinç Kutlutürkan, and Murat Korkmaz. "The Effect of Aromatherapy Massage on Knee Pain and Functional Status in Participants with Osteoarthritis." *Pain Management Nursing* 20, no. 1 (February 2019): 62–69. doi:10.1016/j.pmn.2017.12.001.

Ballard, Clive G., John T. O'Brien, Katharina Reichelt, and Elaine K. Perry. "Aromatherapy as a Safe and Effective Treatment for the Management of Agitation in Severe Dementia: The Results of a Double-Blind, Placebo-Controlled Trial with Melissa." *Journal of Clinical Psychiatry* 63, no. 7 (July 2002): 553–58.

Battaglia, Salvatore. *The Complete Guide to Aromatherapy*. Brisbane, Australia: Watson Ferguson and Co., 2005.

Bliddal, H., A. Rosetzsky , P. Schlinchting, M. S. Weidner, L. A. Andersen, H. H. Ibfelt, K. Christensen, O. N. Jensen, and J. Barslev. "A Randomized Placebo Controlled Cross-Over Study of Ginger Extracts and Ibuprofen in Osteoarthritis." *Osteoarthritis Cartilage* 8, no. 1 (January 2000): 9–12. doi:10.1053/joca.1999.0264.

Bloomfield, S. F., R. Stanwell-Smith, R. W. Crevel, and J. Pickup. "Too Clean, or Not Too Clean: The Hygiene Hypothesis and Home Hygiene." *Clinical & Experimental Allergy* 36, no. 4 (April 2006): 402–25. doi:10.1111/j.1365-2222.2006.02463.x.

Buckle, Jane. *Clinical Aromatherapy in Nursing*. San Diego: Singular Publishing Group, 1997.

Buckle, Jane. *Clinical Aromatherapy: Essential Oils in Healthcare*, 3rd ed. London: Churchill Livingstone, 2015.

Farage, Miranda A., Kenneth W. Miller, Enzo Berardesca, and Howard I. Maibach. "Clinical Implications of Aging Skin." *American Journal of Clinical Dermatology* 10, no. 2 (April 2009): 73–86. doi:10.2165/00128071-200910020-00001.

Field, Tiffany. "Massage Therapy Research Review." *Complementary Therapies in Clinical Practice* 20, no. 4 (November 2014): 224–29. doi:10.1016/j.ctcp.2014.07.002.

Harman, Ann. *Harvest to Hydrosol*. Fruitland, WA: BotANNicals, 2015.

Hoffmann, David. *An Elder's Herbal: Natural Techniques for Promoting Health and Vitality*. Rochester, VT: Healing Arts Press, 1993.

International Federation of Professional Aromatherapists. "Pregnancy Guidelines." Accessed March 28, 2019. https://naha.org/assets/uploads /PregnancyGuidelines-Oct11.pdf.

Lawless, Julia. *The Illustrated Encyclopedia of Essential Oils: A Complete Guide to the Use of Oil in Aromatherapy and Herbalism.* Rockport, MA: Element Books, 1995.

Lundberg, Ulf. "Stress Hormones in Health and Illness: The Roles of Work and Gender." *Psychoneuroendocrinology* 30, no. 10 (November 2005): 1017–21. doi:10.1016/j.psyneuen.2005.03.014.

Mojay, Gabriel. *Aromatherapy for Healing the Spirit: Restoring Emotional and Mental Balance with Essential Oils.* Rochester, VT: Healing Arts Press, 2000.

National Association for Holistic Aromatherapy. "Safety Information." Accessed March 28, 2019. https://naha.org/explore-aromatherapy/safety.

Price, Shirley, and Len Price. *Aromatherapy for Health Professionals*, 4th ed. London: Churchill Livingstone, 2012.

Rhind, Jennifer Peace. *Essential Oils: A Handbook for Aromatherapy Practice,* 2nd ed. London: Singing Dragon, 2012.

Schnaubelt, Kurt. *Medical Aromatherapy: Healing with Essential Oils.* Berkeley: North Atlantic Books, 1999.

Schnaubelt, Kurt. *The Healing Intelligence of Essential Oils: The Science of Advanced Aromatherapy.* Rochester, VT: Healing Arts Press, 2011.

Sherriff, A., A. Farrow, J. Golding, the ALSPAC Study Team, and J. Henderson. "Frequent Use of Chemical Household Products Is Associated with Persistent Wheezing in Pre-school Age Children." *Thorax* 60, no. 1 (January 2005): 45–49. doi:10.1136/thx.2004.021154.

Smith, C. A., C. T. Collins, and C. A. Crowther. "Aromatherapy for Pain Management in Labour." *Cochrane Database of Systematic Reviews*, 2011, no. 7. doi:10.1002/14651858.CD009215.

Tiran, Denise. *Clinical Aromatherapy for Pregnancy and Childbirth.* London: Churchill Livingstone, 2000.

Tiran, Denise. *Aromatherapy in Midwifery Practice.* London: Singing Dragon, 2016.

Tisserand, Robert, and Rodney Young. *Essential Oil Safety*, 2nd ed. London: Churchill Livingstone, 2014.

Worwood, Valerie Ann. *The Fragrant Pharmacy: A Complete Guide to Aromatherapy and Essential Oils.* London: Bantam Books, 1990.

Applications and Recipe Index

Index

Acknowledgments

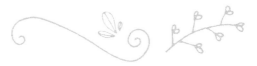

The author would like to acknowledge the significant contribution made to essential oil safety protocols by Rodney Young and Robert Tisserand. Their *Essential Oil Safety (2nd edition)* provides a thorough and balanced approach to assessing existing essential oil safety data. The author would also like to acknowledge and thank Cathy Skipper and Florian Birkmayer of AromaGnosis Online School for their pioneering work with essential oils and aromatherapy as well as their support for and encouragement of the author's contribution to the aromatherapy community. The author would like to acknowledge the following organizations for their hard work and dedication to medicinal and aromatic plant conservation and sustainability: United Plant Savers, the Sustainable Herbs Project, FairWild Foundation, and the IUCN Red List. Thank you all for advocating for the plants and their ecosystems.

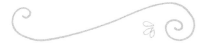

About the Author

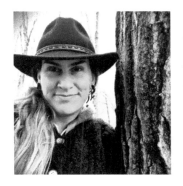

ERIKA GALENTIN, MNIMH, RH (AHG), is a clinical herbalist and an ITEC-certified clinical aromatherapist consulting from Sovereignty Herbs in Athens and Columbus, Ohio. She holds a degree in herbal medicine from the University of Wales, Cardiff, UK, and Scottish School of Herbal Medicine, Glasgow, UK. She is a professional member of the National Institute of Medical Herbalists (UK) and the American Herbalists Guild (USA). She is also a proud member of Pi Alpha Xi National Honor Society in Horticulture (USA). Over a decade of clinical practice has provided a platform for a deep and influential understanding of the efficacy of medicinal plants and essential oils within a clinical environment, and it is through this clinical practice that Erika seeks to encourage positive, learned, and respectful relationships between plants and people. She grows and distills aromatic plants for Sovereignty Herbs from her homestead in southeastern Ohio.

CPSIA information can be obtained
at www.ICGtesting.com
Printed in the USA
BVHW061728240719
554264BV00001B/1

9 781641 525114